汉英对照

中医养生经典译丛
Chinese-English Translation of Traditional Chinese Medicine Classics on Health Preservation

养老奉亲书

The Book for Longevity of Supporting Aged Relatives

[宋] 陈直 撰

范延妮 韩辉 主译

山东科学技术出版社

·济南·

图书在版编目（CIP）数据

养老奉亲书：汉英对照 /（宋）陈直撰；范延妮，韩辉主译 . -- 济南：山东科学技术出版社，2023.3
（2025.3 重印）
（中医养生经典译丛）
ISBN 978-7-5723-1495-7

Ⅰ.①养… Ⅱ.①陈… ②范… ③韩… Ⅲ.①老年人 – 养生（中医）– 中国 – 宋代 – 汉、英 Ⅳ.① R161.7 ② R212

中国国家版本馆 CIP 数据核字 (2023) 第 026540 号

养老奉亲书

YANGLAO FENGQIN SHU

责任编辑：马　祥　夏元枢
装帧设计：孙小杰

主管单位	山东出版传媒股份有限公司
出 版 者	山东科学技术出版社
	地址：济南市市中区舜耕路 517 号
	邮编：250003　电话：（0531）82098088
	网址：www.lkj.com.cn
	电子邮件：sdkj@sdcbcm.com
发 行 者	山东科学技术出版社
	地址：济南市市中区舜耕路 517 号
	邮编：250003　电话：（0531）82098067
印 刷 者	北京兰星球彩色印刷有限公司
	地址：北京市海淀区亮甲店 1 号
	邮编：100020　电话：（010）58411596

规格：16 开（170 mm×240 mm）
印张：15.5　字数：185 千
版次：2023 年 3 月第 1 版　印次：2025 年 3 月第 2 次印刷
定价：78.00 元

译 者

主　译 范延妮　韩　辉
副主译 王芳芳　杨　凡
译　者（以姓氏笔画为序）
　　　　王芳芳　丛正源　杨　凡
　　　　范延妮　韩　辉

丛书序

中医学注重未病先防，倡导不治已病治未病，强调养生的重要性。自《黄帝内经》问世以来，华佗、张仲景、王冰、叶天士等历代医家无不关注养生，或辑先人经验，或创心法要诀，或撰养生精要，护佑中华民族繁衍生息。2021年5月，习近平主席在全球健康峰会上发表题为《携手共建人类卫生健康共同体》的重要讲话，首次提出打造人类卫生健康共同体。中医学作为中华文明的瑰宝，其中凝聚着中华古人智慧的中医养生典籍也应当为全人类健康福祉服务。为此，我们精选《养老奉亲书》《三元参赞延寿书》《养性延命录》《饮膳正要》等经典养生古籍并译为英文，是为"中医养生经典译丛"，以飨读者。

《养老奉亲书》，宋代陈直撰，包括饮食调治、形证脉候、医药扶持、性气好嗜、宴处起居、食治老人诸疾方等内容，主要论述老年保健、四时摄养措施、疾病预防理论及治疗方法，主张老人有病，先食疗之，未愈则命药疗之，饮食宜温热熟饮、忌黏硬生冷，药饵宜用扶持之法，对老年养生具有指导意义。

《三元参赞延寿书》，元代李鹏飞撰，将人之寿命分为天元、地元、人元。"天元之寿"为"精神不耗者得之"，讨论人欲生殖，提出欲不可绝、欲不可早、欲不可纵、欲不可强、欲有所忌、欲有所避等主张；"地元之寿"为"起居有常者得之"，讨论情绪与起居，包括调情绪、慎起居、顺天时等；"人元之寿"为"饮食有度者得之"，讨论健康饮食，提出许多饮食养生方法。

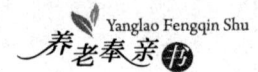

《养性延命录》，南北朝陶弘景撰，辑录上自炎黄、下至魏晋的养生理论与方法，分上、下两卷，包括《教诫篇》《食诫篇》《杂诫忌禳害祈善篇》《服气疗病篇》《导引按摩篇》《御女损益篇》六篇，分别讲述养生理论、饮食宜忌、日常起居、行气之术、导引按摩和房中术，是道教史上对养生术的一次大总结，反映了道教学者对益寿延年的重视。

《饮膳正要》，元代忽思慧撰，是一部营养学专著，共三卷：卷一是诸般禁忌、聚珍异馔；卷二是诸般汤煎、食疗诸病及食物相反中毒等；卷三是米谷品、兽品、禽品、鱼品、果菜品和料物等。内容主要阐述各种饮馔的性味与滋补作用，还包括医疗卫生，历代名医的验方、秘方和具有蒙古族饮食特点的各种肉、乳食品，为我国现存最早的饮食卫生和食疗专书，对研究中医药，尤其是蒙古医药科技史具有重要的意义。

译者团队选取四部典籍的权威版本为蓝本，并参照多个通行本进行校勘，依据世界卫生组织、世界中医药学会联合会等颁布的标准翻译基本名词术语，力争最大限度理解和再现典籍原文内容，为中医海外从业者和研究者开展中医理论溯源和传承创新提供研究基础。

由于译者水平有限，加之时间紧张，错讹之处敬请读者批评指正。

译　者

2023 年 3 月

翻译说明

1. 本次所译的《养老奉亲书》以文津阁钦定四库全书本为汉语底本，并参考了多个通行本。

2. 典籍书名采用音译的方法翻译，音译以词为单位，括号中附以英语翻译。例如《千金翼方》译为 *Qianjin Yifang*（*Supplement to Prescriptions Worth a Thousand Gold Pieces*）。

3. 中草药名称的翻译采取"四保险"的翻译方法，即每个本草名称均按拼音、汉字、英语和拉丁语的方式进行翻译，拉丁语根据世界中医药学会联合会制定的《中医基本名词术语中英对照国际标准》进行翻译，例如"地黄"译为 Dihuang［地黄，Rehmannia Root, Rehmanniae Radix］。方剂名称，采取拼音加英文的方法翻译。

4. 部分原书内容封建迷信内容较多，与医学关系不大，如"贫富祸福第六"，后人在校注本中或删除或移至文末。为保持书籍原貌，本书未做改动，供读者辨别查阅。

5. 书中涉及的药物剂量单位属宋代度量衡单位，与现代度量衡单位有别，均采用音译方法，基本形式和释义如下。

传统剂量单位	公制剂量单位	音译形式
分	0.639 克	Fen
钱	6.389 克	Qian
两	63.888 克	Liang
斤	1 022.208 克	Jin
合	66 毫升	He
升	660 毫升	Sheng
斗	6 600 毫升	Dou
寸	3.168 厘米	Cun

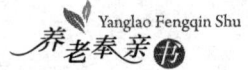

Translation Specification

1. The translation of *Yanglao Fengqin Shu*（*The Book for Longevity of Supporting Aged Relatives*）takes its Chinese photocopy from the *Complete Library in the Four Branches of Literature* stored in Wenjin Chamber as the master copy, and also refers to many current versions.

2. Name of ancient books is transliterated from Chinese character into Pinyin in phrases with the English version in bracket. For instance, *Qianjin Yifang*（*Supplement to Prescriptions Worth a Thousand Gold Pieces*）. Formula names are translated with Pinyin and English in bracket.

3. For the translation of herbal names, the "Four Assurance Method" is adopted, namely, every herbal name is translated in the way that its 4 forms are listed in the sequence of Pinyin, Chinese character, English and Latin. Latin is decided by *International Standard Chinese-English Basic Nomendature of Chinese Medicine* published by World Federation of Chinese Medine Societies. For instance, "地黄" is translated into Dihuang ［地黄, Rehmannia Root, Rehmanniae Radix］.

4. Some of the contents in this book, which are likely to be considered superstitious or irrelevant with medicine such as *Chapter 6 Poverty, Richness, Weal and Woe*, are removed or moved to the end of the book by different collators in later generations. To retain and present the original state honestly, this book made no revision of these contents and the readers are supposed to differentiate themselves.

5. The dosage units involved in this book is in accordance with those in Song Dynasty, quite different with modern ones, so they are transliterated into Pinyin. Refer to the table below.

Traditional dosage unit	Metric dosage unit	Pinyin
分	0.639 g	Fen
钱	6.389 g	Qian
两	63.888 g	Liang
斤	1 022.208 g	Jin
合	66 mL	He
升	660 mL	Sheng
斗	6 600 mL	Dou
寸	3.168 cm	Cun

本书为山东中医药大学英语专业建设成果；山东中医药大学"中医话语特征与中医翻译"青年科研创新团队成果；山东中医药大学中医养生学学科建设与专业建设成果。

目 录

Contents

饮食调治第一

Chapter 1　Health Cultivation with Proper Diet ………… 001

形证脉候第二

Chapter 2　Identification of Body, Syndrome, and Pulse Patterns

……………………………………………………… 005

医药扶持第三

Chapter 3　Medicinal Support ………………………… 008

性气好嗜第四

Chapter 4　Temperaments and Hobbies ……………… 011

宴处起居第五

Chapter 5　Daily Routine About Shelter and Living Conditions

……………………………………………………… 014

贫富祸福第六

Chapter 6　Poverty, Richness, Weal and Woe ………… 017

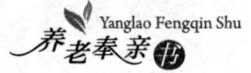

戒忌保护第七
Chapter 7　Precautions and Taboos ················· 020

四时养老总序第八
Chapter 8　Methods to Support the Aged in the Four Seasons ············ 023
　　四时通用男女妇人方
　　General Formulas for Women and Men in the Four Seasons ·········· 025

春时摄养第九
Chapter 9　Health Preservation in Spring ················ 051
　　春时用诸药方
　　Formulas for the Aged in Spring ················ 054

夏时摄养第十
Chapter 10　Health Preservation in Summer ················ 061
　　夏时用药诸方
　　Formulas for the Aged in Summer ················ 064

秋时摄养第十一
Chapter 11　Health Preservation in Autumn ················ 076
　　秋时用药诸方
　　Formulas for the Aged in Autumn ················ 078

冬时摄养第十二
Chapter 12　Health Preservation in Winter ················ 085
　　冬时用药诸方
　　Formulas for the Aged in Winter ················ 087

食治养老序第十三

Chapter 13　Preface to the Support of the Aged with Diet Therapy
·· 090

食治老人诸疾方第十四

Chapter 14　Formulas to Treat Various Diseases of the Aged with Diet Therapy
·· 094

食治养老益气方

Formulas to Support the Aged and Benefit Qi with Diet Therapy ··· 094

增补方剂

Supplementary Formulas ·· 101

食治眼目方

Formulas to Treat Eye Diseases of the Aged with Diet Therapy
·· 104

增补方剂

Supplementary Formulas ·· 110

食治耳聋耳鸣诸方

Formulas to Treat Deaf and Tinnitus of the Aged with Diet Therapy
·· 111

增补方剂

Supplementary Formulas ·· 115

食治五劳七伤诸方

Formulas to Treat Five Kinds of Consumptive Diseases and Seven Damages of the Aged with Diet Therapy ·················· 115

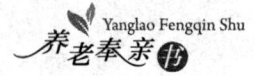

增补方剂

Supplementary Formulas ································ 119

食治虚损羸瘦诸方

Formulas to Treat Deficiency and Emaciation of the Aged with Diet Therapy ································ 122

增补方剂

Supplementary Formulas ································ 126

食治脾胃气弱方

Formulas to Treat Qi Deficiency of the Spleen and the Stomach of the Aged with Diet Therapy ································ 127

增补方剂

Supplementary Formulas ································ 134

食治泻痢诸方

Formulas to Treat Diarrhea of the Aged with Diet Therapy ·········· 136

增补方剂

Supplementary Formulas ································ 143

食治烦渴热诸方

Formulas to Treat Vexation, Thirst, and Fever of the Aged with Diet Therapy ································ 145

增补方剂

Supplementary Formulas ································ 152

食治水气诸方

Formulas to Treat Edema Disease of the Aged with Diet Therapy ································ 153

食治喘嗽诸方

Formulas to Treat Panting and Cough of the Aged with Diet Therapy
·· 159

增补方剂

Supplementary Formulas ················· 167

食治脚气诸方

Formulas to Treat Beriberi of the Aged with Diet Therapy ········ 170

增补方剂

Supplementary Formulas ················· 177

食治诸淋方

Formulas to Treat Stranguria of the Aged with Diet Therapy········ 178

增补方剂

Supplementary Formulas ················· 184

食治噎塞诸方

Formulas to Treat Dysphagia of the Aged with Diet Therapy ······ 185

食治冷气诸方

Formulas to Treat Cold Syndrome of the Aged with Diet Therapy
·· 191

增补方剂

Supplementary Formulas ················· 197

食治诸痔方

Formulas to Treat Hemorrhoids of the Aged with Diet Therapy
·· 198

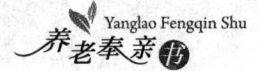

增补方剂

Supplementary Formulas ································· 204

食治诸风方

Formulas to Treat Wind Syndrome of the Aged with Diet Therapy
·· 205

简妙老人备急方

Simple and Effective Formulas for Emergency of the Aged ········· 216

养老奉亲书续添

Supplementation ································· 229

饮食调治第一

Chapter 1　Health Cultivation with Proper Diet

主身者神，养气者精，益精者气，资气者食，食者生民之天，活人之本也，故饮食进则谷气充，谷气充则气血胜，气血胜则筋力强。故脾胃者，五脏之宗也。四脏之气，皆禀于脾，故四时皆以胃气为本。《生气通天论》云：气味，辛甘发散为阳，酸苦涌泄为阴。是以一身之中，阴阳运用，五行相生，莫不由于饮食也。

It is the spirit that governs the body, the essence that nourishes the qi, the qi that benefits the essence, and the food that supports qi. Food is the first necessity and the essential of man. Therefore, food provides sufficient nutrient essence, which further supplements qi and blood, and the vigorous qi and blood further strengthen tendons and muscles. Thus the spleen and stomach rank top in the five zang-organs. As the spleen qi benefits qi of the other 4 zang-organs, stomach qi is regarded as primary in the four seasons. *Shengqi Tongtian Lun* (*Discussion on the Interrelationship Between Life and Nature*) says: In terms of flavors, pungent and sweet flavors pertain to yang because they disperse, while sour and bitter flavors pertain to yin because they induce vomiting and purgation. Thus the movement and transformation between yin and yang and generation among the five elements in the body are all related with the diet.

若少年之人，真元气壮，或失于饥饱，食于生冷，以根本强盛，未易为患。其高年之人，真气耗竭，五脏衰弱，全仰饮食以资气血。若生冷无节，饥饱失宜，调停无度，动成疾患。

For the young people who have sufficient vitality, they may suffer from hunger and satiation or take cold or raw food, but they are not susceptible to diseases due to their vigorous constitution. However, for the aged, they are deficient in essential qi and weak in the five zang-organs, so they depend wholly on the diet to nourish the qi and blood. If they take cold or raw food inordinately, or suffer from hunger and satiation, or get excessive recuperation, they tend to be sick.

凡人疾病，未有不因八邪而感。所谓八邪者，风、寒、暑、湿、饥、饱、劳、逸也。为人子者，得不慎之。

All the diseases are believed to be caused by 8 kinds of pathogenic factors, namely wind, cold, summer-heat, dampness, hunger, satiety, fatigue, and leisure. Therefore, people should take these factors into consideration and take care of their parents cautiously.

若有疾患，且先详食医之法，审其疾状，以食疗之。食疗未愈，然后命药，贵不伤其脏腑也。

凡百饮食，必在人子躬亲调治，无纵婢使慢其所食。

If the aged get ill, it is advised to consult the dietician first and treat them with dietotherapy based on their syndrome and symptoms. If this does not work, medicinal method can be used then to avoid the damage to their zang-fu organs.

All kinds of foods should be prepared by the children of the aged themselves instead of the servants to reduce impropriety.

老人之食，大抵宜其温热熟软，忌其粘硬生冷。每日晨朝，宜以醇酒，先进平补下元药一服，女人则平补血海药一服，无燥热者良。寻以猪、羊肾粟米粥一杯呷之，五味、葱、薤、鹑臇等粥皆可。至辰时，服人参平胃散一服，然后次第以顺四时软熟饮食进之。食后，引行一二百步，令运动消散。临卧时，进化痰利膈人参半夏丸一服。

In general, the foods for the aged ought to be warm, hot, cooked and soft, while those that are sticky, hard, raw and cold should be forbidden. Every morning, the old man can take one dose of medicine to tonify the lower energizer with mellow wine, while the old woman can take one dose of medicine to nourish blood. It should be ensured that no dryness-heat symptom occurs after taking the doses. Before long they can take some millet porridge mixed with pork or goat kidney, or porridge mixed with 5 kinds of seasonings, scallion, Chinese chive, quail spine, etc. When it comes to 7 to 9 o'clock in the morning, they can take one dose of Renshen Pingwei San （Stomach-Calming Powder added with Ginseng）, then take some soft and cooked foods that correspond to the four seasons in order. After dinner, they had better walk for 100 to 200 steps accompanied by others to help digestion. When they are prepared to go to bed, they can take one dose of Renshen Banxia Wan (Ginseng and Pinellia Pill), which is effective to transform phlegm and disinhibit the diaphragm.

尊年之人，不可顿饱，但频频与食，使脾胃易化，谷气长存。若顿令饱食，则多伤满，缘衰老人肠胃虚薄，不能消纳，故成疾患。为人子者，深宜体悉，此养老人之大要也。

For the aged, it is suggested to have proper amount of food frequently instead of very full meals one time to relieve the burden of the spleen and stomach, and protect the essence derived from food. If they take a lot at one meal, it may impair the intestines and stomach and cause abnormal distention and fullness. That is because their intestines and stomach are too weak to digest and absorb too much food, which may result in diseases finally. For those who have elderly parents, they should experience and perceive that in person for that is the key point to support the aged.

日止可进前药三服，不可多饵。如无疾患，亦不须服药，但只调停饮食，自然无恙矣。

Three doses of the medicinals mentioned above can be taken a day but no more than that is advised. If there is no diseases, the medicinals are not necessary. The proper diet will keep the disease away.

形证脉候第二

Chapter 2　Identification of Body, Syndrome, and Pulse Patterns

　　《上古天真论》曰：女子之数七，丈夫之数八。女子七七四十九，任脉虚，冲脉衰，天癸竭，地道不通。丈夫八八六十四，五脏皆衰，筋骨懈堕，天癸尽，脉弱形枯。女子过六十之期，丈夫逾七十之年，越天常数。上寿之人，若衣食丰备，子孙勤养，承顺慈亲，参行孝礼，能调其饮食，适其寒温，上合神灵，下契人理，此顺天之道也。

　　Shanggu Tianzhen Lun（Ancient Ideas on How to Preserve Natural Healthy） indicates: 7 is a lesser yang number for women who pertain to yin, and thus it is a custom to count woman's age by 7. 8 is a lesser yin number for men who pertain to yang, and thus it is a custom to count man's age by 8. In this way, yin within yang and yang within yin are accomplished. For women, when they reach 49（7 times 7）years old, their conception vessel and thoroughfare vessel become deficient, and their reproduction-stimulating essence is also exhausted, which lead to the stagnation of female genital duct. For men, when they reach 64（8 times 8）years old, their five zang-organs are exhausted, sinews and bones are drooped, reproduction-stimulating essence is also exhausted, pulse is weak and thus their bodies are withered. If the age of women exceeds 60 and the age of men exceeds 70, they will be considered to break the law of nature. The longevous are usually supported sufficiently, served cautiously, respected obediently, loved amiably, and treated with filial piety by their offspring. Their diet should be properly prepared and served at comfortable temperature. Their life corresponds to the nature and the society perfectly, and this is what we call conforming to the law of nature.

高年之人，形羸气弱，理自当然。其有丈夫、女子年逾七十，面色红润，形气康强，饮食不退，尚多秘热者，此理何哉？且年老之人，痿瘁为常，今反此者，非真阳血海气壮也？但诊左右手脉，须大紧数，此老人延永之兆也。老人真气已衰，此得虚阳气盛，充于肌体，则两手脉大，饮食倍进，双脸常红，精神强健，此皆虚阳气所助也。须时有烦渴膈热，大腑秘结，但随时以平常汤药，微微消解，三五日间自然平复。常得虚阳气存，自然饮食得进，此天假其寿也。切不得为有小热，频用转泻之药通利，苦冷之药疏解。若虚阳气退，复归真体，则形气尪羸，脏腑衰弱，多生冷疾，无由补复。

It is normal for the aged to have weak physique and deficient qi. There are some old men and women whose age is over 70, having rosy complexion, strong physique, vigorous qi, good appetite, but constipation due to heat. How come? The aged usually present a poor physique and weak muscles and tendons. Therefore, for those who present the opposite features, do they really have such strong kidney yang and vigorous qi in the thoroughfare vessel?

When examining their pulses on the left and right hands, their pulses are powerful, tight and rapid, which is a sign of longevity. Since the genuine qi of the aged has been exhausted, this condition is the result of qi exuberance due to false yang, manifested as surging pulse, doubled appetite, rosy complexion and high spirit. All of these signs are actually induced by false yang in the body. Sometimes symptoms like vexation, thirst, diaphragm heat, stagnation of the large intestine and constipation may occur, which can be relieved in several days by taking some ordinary decoctions. The long existence of false yang and vigorous qi will improve the appetite, which is the extra longevity granted by nature. Therefore, the frequent use of purging medicinal to defecate, bitter and cold medicinal to discharge should be forbidden when treating slight heat of the aged. When the false yang disappears, the actual state of physique will come back such as weak body, qi, and zang-fu organs, and cold syndrome, which can not be restored in any way.

若是从来无虚阳之气，一向惫乏之人，全在斟量汤剂，常加温补，调停粥，以为养治，此养老之先也。

For people who have no false yang, they may feel lassitude and tired all along. The proper decoction, warming and tonifying medicinals, and thick porridge can be used to cultivate their health, which is the priority of supporting the aged.

医药扶持第三

Chapter 3　Medicinal Support

　　常见世人治高年之人疾患，将同年少，乱投汤药，妄行针灸，以攻其疾，务欲速愈。殊不知上寿之人，血气已衰，精神减耗，危若风烛，百疾易攻。至于视听不至聪明，手足举动不随，其身体劳倦，头目昏眩，风气不顺，宿疾时发，或秘或泄，或冷或热，此皆老人之常态也。不顺治之，紧用针药，务求痊瘥，往往因此别致危殆。且攻病之药，或吐，或汗，或解，或利。缘衰老之人，不同年少，真气壮盛，虽汗吐转利，未至危困。其老弱之人，若汗之则阳气泄，吐之则胃气逆，泻之则元气脱，立致不虞，此养老之大忌也。

　　It is common to see physicians treat the aged as the young by randomly adopting decoction and acupuncture and moxibustion, hoping to cure the disease as soon as possible. The fact has been neglected that the aged, like a candle in the wind, are very weak in blood and qi, exhausted in the essence and spirit, and susceptible to all kinds of diseases. The followings are ordinary symptoms of the aged—declining of vision and hearing, difficult movement of hands and feet, fatigue of body, dizziness, abnormal flow of qi, intermittent bursts of inveterate diseases, constipation or diarrhea, and cold or heat. If the treatment does not follow the way suitable for the aged, and applies acupuncture and medicinals immediately in order to cure completely, it may arouse other dangerous pathogenic factors. Furthermore, the medicinals are often used to treat diseases by vomiting, sweating, discharging or purging. The aged are different from the young who have strong genuine qi. For the young, the method of vomiting, sweating and discharging may not cause dangerous situation. For the aged, the sweating method will cause the discharge of yang qi; the vomiting method will lead to the counter-flow of stomach qi; the purging method will exhaust original qi. The unexpected thing tends to be incurred quickly at any time, which should be forbidden in supporting the aged.

大体老人药饵，止是扶持之法。只可用温平顺气，进食补虚中和之药治之，不可用市肆赎买，他人惠送，不知方味，及野狼虎之药，与之服饵，切宜审详。若身有宿疾，或时发动，则随其疾状，用中和汤药，顺三朝五日，自然无事。然后调停饮食，依食医之法，随食性变馔治之，此最为良也。

Generally speaking, drugs administered to the aged should follow the method of supporting. Only the medicinals with warm and mild properties, tonifying and moderating functions can be used. The medicinals bought or redeemed from the market, given by others, unknown of ingredients, or thought to be of strong and drastic properties must be examined carefully when used to the aged. When the inveterate disease occurs, some harmonizing decoction can be used according to the symptom. Up to 3 to 5 days, the disease will be cured. Then the diet can be adjusted according to the method suggested by dietician, diversified and prepared in accordance with the nature of food, which will be the best way to support the aged.

性气好嗜第四

Chapter 4　Temperaments and Hobbies

眉寿之人，形气虽衰，心亦自壮，但不能遂时人事遂其所欲。虽居温给，亦常不足，故多咨煎背执，等闲喜怒，性气不定，止如小儿。全在承顺颜色，遂其所欲，严戒婢使子孙，不令违背。若愤怒一作，血气虚弱，中气不顺，因而饮食，便成疾患。深宜体悉。

　　The aged with long brow are weak in physique and qi but their thoughts are still active. They can not always have their wishes fulfilled with their own efforts following the changing of time and human relationship. Although they are well accommodated with food and clothes, they often feel unsatisfied. Therefore, they often sigh, feel anxious, look obstinate, show unreasonable joy or anger and act temperamentally just like children. It is all up to their children to cater to their aged and do as what they wish. It is forbidden for their children and servants to disobey the aged. If the aged are irritated, they are likely to get weak in blood and qi and stagnated in middle energizer. In this case, the food they take in may not be digested as usual and even lead to disorders. People should put themselves into their parents' shoes when taking care of them.

常令人随侍左右，不可令孤坐独寝。缘老人孤僻，易于伤感，才觉孤寂，便生郁闷。养老之法，凡人平生为性，各有好嗜之事，见即喜之。有好书画者，有好琴棋者，有好赌扑者，有好珍奇者，有好药饵者，有好禽鸟者，有好古物者，有好佛事者，有好丹灶者。人之僻好，不能备举，但以其平生偏嗜之物，时为寻求，择其精绝者，布于左右，使其喜爱，玩悦不已，老人衰倦，无所用心。若只令守家孤坐，自成滞闷。今见所好之物，自然用心于物上，日自看承戏玩，自以为乐，虽有劳倦，咨煎性气，自然减可。

The aged had better be accompanied and served by servants instead of being left seated alone or sleeping alone. That is because the aged tend to be unsociable, sentimental and solitary, which may cause depression. The way to support the aged should be closely related to their physiological characteristics formed throughout their life, because everyone has his own special hobby which makes him happy. There is someone who likes painting and calligraphy, someone who likes musical instrument and chess, someone who likes gambling, someone who likes rare treasure, someone who likes elixir, someone who likes birds, someone who likes antiques, someone who likes Buddhist ceremony, and someone who likes alchemy to refine pills of immortality. It is hard to list all the special hobbies of human beings. However, when the favorite thing of the aged is hunted out and the delicate one is chosen and placed around them now and again in order to please them, they will indulge themselves in the presents without thinking about other things as they have no extra energy. Otherwise, they may feel depressed and dull if being left alone at home. The aged will put their mind into the likings that are available. To observe and play their favourite possession will be their daily job, which will bring them great pleasure. In this way, the previous fatigue, sigh and odd temperament will be relieved naturally.

宴处起居第五

Chapter 5　Daily Routine About Shelter and Living Conditions

凡人衰晚之年，心力倦怠，精神耗短，百事懒于施为，盖气血筋力之使然也。全藉子孙孝养，竭力将护，以免非横之虞。凡行住坐卧，宴处起居，皆须巧立制度，以助娱乐。

When people get old, they tend to feel lassitude. Due to the exhaustion of mind and spirit, the aged are reluctant to do anything, which may be resulted from the deficiency of qi, blood, essence and energy. Therefore, it all relies on the children to go all out for supporting and taking care of the aged in case some severe accident should occur. As long as the thing is related to transportation and shelter of the aged, it should be set with regulations thoughtfully in order to please and entertain them.

栖息之室，必常洁雅。夏则虚敞，冬则温密。其寝寐床榻，不须高广，比常之制三分减一，低则易于升降，狭则不容漫风。裀褥厚藉，务在软平。三面设屏，以防风冷。其枕宜用夹熟色帛为之，实以菊花，制在低，则寝无罅风，长则转不落枕。其所坐椅，宜作矮禅床样，坐可垂足履地，易于兴起。左右置栏，面前设几。缘老多困，坐则成眠，有所栏围，免闪侧之伤。

The living room of the aged should always be clean and elegant. In summer, the room should be spacious and ventilated. In winter, it should be kept warm and wind-tight. The bed of the aged need not be tall and broad, usually one third lower than the normal one in height. The lower height makes it easy for the aged to go to bed and get out of bed. The narrower size keeps the aged away from draught. Put double layered mattress, cotton-padded mattress, and straw mattress on the bed. Make sure it is soft and flat. Set screens around the bed to prevent cold wind. The pillow should better be made by boiled colorful silk with Juhua［菊花，Chrysanthemums, Chrysanthemi Flos］inside. The size of it should be thin and long, preventing wind from the gap between pillow and bed, and stiff neck when turning the head. The chair should better be as high as the square meditating stool, which makes it easy for the feet to reach the ground, and to stand up. Set bars on the left and right side of the chair and short table in front of it. That is because the aged tend to feel sleepy and even take a nap when they are seated. In this situation, the bars can protect them from sprain caused by turning around or toppling.

其衣服制度，不须宽长。长则多有蹶绊，宽则衣服不著身。缘老人骨肉疏冷，风寒易中，若窄衣贴身，暖气著体，自然血气流利，四肢和畅。虽遇盛夏，亦不可令袒露。其颈后连项，常用紫软夹帛，自颈后巾帻中垂下著肉，入衣领中至背甲间，以护腠理。尊年人肌肉瘦怯，腠理开疏，若风伤腠中，便成大患，深宜慎之。

Their clothes need not be too loose and long. If they are too long, tottering or toppling is likely to take place. If they are too loose, they can not fit well. The aged are characterized by bone rarefaction, so they are susceptible to wind-cold. If their clothes fit well and keep them warm, the blood and qi will flow smoothly and the limbs will remain warm and comfortable. Even in midsummer, bareness for the aged should be avoided. The silk padded with arnebia root is usually put around the neck of the aged, hanging from back of the neck down to the back, entering from collar to shoulder blade to protect the interstices. The muscles of the aged are emaciated and flabby, and their interstices are loose. If they are attacked by the wind pathogen, severe disorders may occur, so it should be taken seriously.

贫富祸福第六

Chapter 6　Poverty, Richness, Weal and Woe

《经》曰：自天子至于庶人，孝无终始，而患不及者，未之有也。人子以纯孝之心，竭力事亲，无终始不及之理，惟供养之有厚薄，由贫富之有分限。人居富贵，有奉于己而薄于亲者，人所不录，天所不容，虽处富贵而即贫贱也。人虽居贫贱，能约于己而丰于亲者，人所推仰，天所助与，虽处贫贱而即富贵也。作善降之百祥，作不善降之百殃。善莫大于孝，孝感于天，故天与之福，所以虽贫贱而即富贵也。罪莫大于不孝，不孝感于天，故天与之祸，所以虽富贵而即贫贱也。善恶之报，其犹影响，为人子者，可不信乎？

Jing（*The Classic of Filial Piety*）says: From emperor to common people, no one can escape from misfortune if he doesn't abide by the filial duty constantly. With sincere filial piety, children do their utmost to take care of their parents, so it is hard to say whether they have done it thoroughly or sufficiently. But the difference in supporting the aged can be found between the poor and the rich. People who are wealthy, generous to themselves but mean to their aged relatives, will never be accepted and respected by the

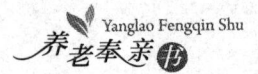

public and the heaven. Though they are rich in wealth, they are indeed poor and lowly in nature. People who are poor though, mean to themselves but generous to their aged relatives, will be admired and aided by the public and the heaven. Though they are poor in wealth, they are indeed wealthy and honorable in nature. Doing good will bring about hundreds of auspiciousness, and doing bad will bring about hundreds of disasters. In terms of goodness, nothing is greater than filial piety. Heaven can sense filial piety, so it will be blessed by heaven, which explains why those people who are poor though, are rich indeed. In terms of crime, nothing is greater than filial impiety. Heaven can sense filial impiety, so it will be cursed by heaven, which explains why those people who are rich though, are poor indeed. The son of the aged should believe the retribution of good and evil, and the influence especially, shouldn't he?

奉亲之道，亦不在日用三牲，但能承顺父母颜色，尽其孝心，随其所有，此顺天之理也。其温厚之家，不可慢于老者，尽依养老之方，励力行之。其贫下阙乏之家，养老之法，虽有奉行之心，而无奉行之力者，但随家丰俭，竭力于亲，约礼设具，使老者知其罄力事奉而止。将见孝心感格，阴灵默佑，如姜诗之跃鲤，孟宗之泣笋，无非孝感所致。此行孝之明验也。

The way of supporting the aged is not necessarily to treat them with sumptuous food such as beef, mutton and pork in daily life, but to obey and please the parents, do the filial piety, and let them own what they wish. This is also following the principle of heaven. The wealthy family should attach importance to the supporting of the aged by striving to follow the health-cultivating methods for the aged; the poor family, with the mind but not enough material conditions to support the aged, should try their best to show filial obedience in accordance with their budget, making proper arrangements for rituals and equipment to let the aged know that they have made best endeavors to serve. Heaven may be moved by the filial piety, and it may be blessed by the deities. Famous legends have shown us filial piety can move heaven, like Jiang Shi's leaping carp and Meng Zong's weeping to bamboo （2 legends in *Chinese Twenty Four Stories of Filial Piety*）. They are cases in point to show the reward for conducting filial piety.

虑孝子顺孙，有窘乏不能依此法者，意有不足，故立此贫富祸福之说以齐之。

It is concerned about people who have filial piety to their aged relatives but cannot follow this method due to poor situation. This chapter is written to encourage them to learn from good examples.

戒忌保护第七

Chapter 7　Precautions and Taboos

人，万物中一物也，不能逃天地之数。若天癸数穷，则精血耗竭，神气浮弱，返同小儿，全假将护以助衰晚。

It is hardly possible for a man to escape from the fate given by heaven as he or she is just one member in the universe. If the amount of reproduction-stimulating essence is diminished, the essence and blood will be exhausted, the spirit will be deficient, and the state of the aged will return to that of child. It is totally relying on other people's care and support to spend the declining years.

若遇水火、兵寇、非横惊怖之事，必先扶侍老人，于安稳处避之，不可喧忙惊动。尊年之人，一遭大惊，便致冒昧，因生余疾。凡丧葬凶祸，不可令吊。疾病危困，不可令惊。悲哀忧愁，不可令人预报。秽恶臭败，不可令食。粘硬毒物，不可令飡。敝漏卑湿，不可令居。猝风暴寒，不可令冒。烦暑燠热，不可令中。动作行步，不可令劳。暮夜之食，不可令饱。阴雾晦暝，不可令饥。假借鞍马，不可令乘。偏僻药饵，不可令服。废宅敧宇，不可令入。坟园冢墓，不可令游。危险之地，不可令行。涧渊之水，不可令渡。暗昧之室，不可令孤。凶祸远报，不可令知。轻薄婢使，不可令亲。家缘冗事，不可令管。

In the event of flood, fire, war, robbery, or other terrible things, the aged must be first moved to a safe place without being annoyed by noise and hurry. The reason is that the aged are easy to be shocked into a trance which may lead to other diseases. Do not let the aged condole in the funerals and misfortunes. Do not let the aged feel startled in diseases and plight. Do not let the aged know sad and sorrow news. Do not let the aged take dirty, smelly or rotten food. Do not let the aged take sticky, hard, or poisonous thing. Do not let the aged live in the dilapidated, leaking, or wet house especially that in a low position. Do not let the aged bear sudden wind and severe cold. Do not let the aged have heatstroke and dysphoria. Do not let the aged feel fatigued in action and walking. Do not let the aged feel satiated in supper. Do not let the aged feel hungry in foggy and cloudy day. Do not let the aged take carriage pulled by borrowed horses. Do not let the aged take medicine made in remote areas. Do not let the aged live in deserted house or house with its eaves collapsed. Do not let the aged visit graveyard. Do not let the aged walk in dangerous places. Do not let the aged cross deep stream in chasms. Do not let the aged stay alone in dusky room. Do not let the aged know misfortunes sent from far afield. Do not let the aged stay intimate with the female servant who is dissolute. Do not let the aged manage complicated and trivial family affairs.

若此事类颇多，不克备举。但人子悉意深虑，过为之防，稍不便于老人者，皆宜忌之，以保长年。常宜游息精蓝，崇尚佛事，使神识趣向，一归善道，此养老之奇术也。

There are so many things of this kind that it is impossible to list them all here. People should be cautious and thoughtful to take precautions against unexpected incidents for their aged relatives. Anything that is inconvenient for the aged should be avoided to ensure their longevity. It is recommended for the aged to visit beautiful places with excellent environment and focus on Buddhist service to orient the spirit and interest to charitable things, which is also an effective way to preserve health.

四时养老总序第八

Chapter 8　Methods to Support the Aged in the Four Seasons

《四时调神论》曰：阴阳四时者，万物之终始，死生之本也。逆之则灾害生，从之则苛疾不起，是谓得道。春温以生之，夏热以长之，秋凉以收之，冬寒以藏之，若气反于时，则皆为疾疠，此天之常道也，顺之则生，逆之则病。《经》曰：观天之道，执天之行，尽矣。人能执天道生杀之理，法四时运用而行，自然疾病不生，长年可保。

Sishi Tiaoshen Lun（Major Discussion on Regulation of Spirit According to the Changes of the Four Seasons） says: The changes of yin and yang in the four seasons are responsible for the growth, decline and death of all things. Violation of it brings about disasters while abidance by it prevents the occurrence of disasters. This is what to follow the law of nature means. It is warm in spring so everything generates, heat in summer so everything grows, cool in autumn so everything harvests, and cold in winter so everything stores. If the qi turns against the time, disease and plague may occur, which is the law of nature. Following the law ensures life while violating it leads to disease. *Jing（Huangdi's Canon of Implicit*

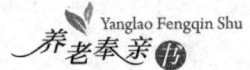

Conjunction）says: To observe the law of nature and behave correspondingly will help extend life span of people to its extreme. If people can adhere to the law of nature, balance yin and yang, follow the principle of health cultivation in the four seasons, they would remain healthy and enjoy longevity.

其黄发之人，五脏气虚，精神耗竭，若稍失节宣，即动成危瘵。盖老人倦惰，不能自调，在人资养以延遐算。为人子者，深宜察其寒温，审其药，依四时摄养之方，顺五行休旺之气，恭恪奉亲，慎无懈怠。今集老人四时通用备疾药法，具陈于左。此方多用寒药，盖北人所宜。凡用药者，宜参处之。

The aged are characterized by qi deficiency in the five zang-organs and exhaustion of essence and spirit. The absence of moderation and regulation may result in severe diseases. It is probably because the aged are tired and indolent and unable to adjust themselves well. They rely on assistance and support from others to realize their longevity. Those who have elderly parents should check their temperature, examine their porridge and medicine, conform to the prescriptions in accordance with the four seasons, follow the law of the five elements dominating corresponding seasons, be respectful and cautious to care the aged without sluggishness. General methods to support the aged with medicinals in the four seasons are collected and stated in this chapter. The medicinals used in these prescriptions are mostly cold in nature, which are more suitable for people in northern China. Those who use these formulas should differentiate syndromes and make proper decision.

四时通用男女妇人方

General Formulas for Women and Men in the Four Seasons

治老人风热上攻，头旋运闷，喜卧，怔悸，起即欲倒，背急身强。旋覆花散。女人通用。

Xuanfuhua San（Inula Flower Powder）is used to treat the aged with symptoms of dizziness, depression, preference to lying, palpitation, tending to fall when getting up, stiff back and body due to wind-heat attacking the head. It is applicable for women.

旋覆花半两　前胡一两　麦门冬一两，去心　蔓荆子半两　白术二分　枳壳二分，去瓤，麸炒　甘菊花三分　半夏半两，姜汁煮　防风半两　大黄虚人宜用石膏　独活半两　甘草半两

It is composed of 0.5 Liang of Xuanfuhua ［旋覆花, Inula Flower, Flos Inula Japonica］, 1 Liang of Qianhu ［前胡, Radix Peucedani, Peucedanum Praeruptorum Dunn］, 1 Liang of Maimendong ［麦门冬, Radix Ophiopogonis, Ophiopogon japonicus Ker-Gawl］ with the core removed, 0.5 Liang of Manjingzi ［蔓荆子, Shrub Chastetree Fruit, Fructus Viticis］, 2 Fen of Baizhu ［白术, Argehead Atractylodes Rhizome, Rhizoma Atractylodis Macrocephalae］, 2 Fen of Zhiqiao ［枳壳, Orange Fruit, Fructus Aurantii］ stir-fried with bran after the pulp being removed, 3 Fen of Ganjuhua ［甘菊花, Chrysanthemum, Chrysanthemi Flos］, 0.5 Liang of Banxia ［半夏, Pinellia Tuber, Rhizoma Pinelliae］ boilt with ginger juice, 0.5 Liang of Fangfeng ［防风, Divaricate

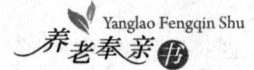

Saposhnikovia Root, Radix Saposhnikoviae], Dahuang［大黄, Rhubarb, Rhei Radix Et Rhizoma］ for common people or Shigao ［石膏, Gypsum, Gypsum Fibrosum］ for those with deficiency; 0.5 Liang of Duhuo ［独活, Pubescent Angelica, Radix Angelicae Pubescentis], 0.5 Liang of Gancao［甘草, Liquorice Root, Radix Glycyrrhizae］.

上为末。每服三钱，水一中盏，入姜半分同煎，至六分，去滓温服，不计时候。

Pound the above ingredients into powder. Take 3 Qian of it each time, put it in a medium cup of water, add half Fen of ginger, decoct it until three fifths is left, take it warm with dregs removed. It can be taken anytime.

老人补壮筋骨，治风走疰疼痛，并风气上攻下疰。羌活丸。

Qianghuo Wan（Notopterygium Pill）is used to strengthen the sinews and bones of the aged, treat the migrating pain caused by wind, and wind pathogen attacking upward and downward.

羌活　牛膝酒浴过，焙干　川楝子　白附子　舶上茴香　黄芪去皮锉　青盐　巴戟去心　黑附子炮制，去皮脐　沙苑　白蒺藜

The pill is composed of Qianghuo ［羌活, Incised Notopterygium Rhizome and Root, Rhizoma et Radix Notopterygii], Niuxi ［牛膝, Twotoothed Achyranthes Root, Radix Achyranthis Bidentatae] dried after being bathed in liquor, Chuanlianzi ［川楝子, Szechwan Chinaberry Fruit, Fructus Meliae Toosendan], Baifuzi ［白附子, Giant Typhonium Rhizome, Rhizoma Typhonii],

Boshanghuixiang［舶上茴香, Star Anise, Anisi Stellati Fructus］, Huangqi［黄芪, Milkvetch Root, Radix Astragali seu Hedysari］with the skin removed and then filed, Qingyan［青盐, Halite, Halitum］, Baji［巴戟, Morinda Root, Radix Morindae Officinalis］with the core removed, black Fuzi［附子, Prepared Common Monkshood Daughter Root, Radix Aconiti Lateralis Preparata］processed with the skin and umbilicus removed, Shayuan［沙苑, Flatstem Milkvetch Seed, Semen Astragali Complanati］and Baijili［白蒺藜, Puncturevine Caltrop Fruit, Fructus Tribuli］.

上件等分，一处捣罗为末，酒煮面糊为丸，如梧桐子大。每服十丸，空心，临卧盐汤下。看老少，加减服。

Pound the above ingredients with equal amount into powder. Boil it with liquor and flour, then make it into pills as big as firmiana seeds. Take 10 pills each time on an empty stomach. Swallow them with weak brine before going to bed. Modify the formula according to the age of patients.

老人和脾胃气，进饮食，止痰逆，疗腹痛气，调中。木香人参散。男子女人通用。

Muxiang Renshen San（Root of Common Aucklandia and Ginseng Powder）is used to regulate the spleen and stomach qi, increase appetite, stop phlegm and qi counterflow, treat abdominal pain and qi distention. It is suitable for both men and women.

木香半两　人参去芦头，半两　茯苓去黑皮，一分　白术半两，微炒　肉豆蔻去皮，一分　枇杷叶去毛，一分　厚朴去粗皮，姜汁制　丁香半两　藿香叶一分　甘草半两，炙　干姜半两，炮　陈皮半两，汤浸，去瓤

The formula is composed of 0.5 Liang of Muxiang［木香，Root of Common Aucklandia, Radix Aucklandiae］, 0.5 Liang of Renshen［人参，Ginseng, Radix Ginseng］with the top removed, 1 Fen of Fuling［茯苓，Indian Bread, Poria］with its black skin removed, 0.5 Liang of Baizhu［白术，Largehead Atractylodes Rhizome, Rhizoma Atractylodis Macrocephalae］fried slightly, 1 Fen of Roudoukou［肉豆蔻，Nutmeg, Semen Myristicae］with the skin removed, 1 Fen of Pipaye［枇杷叶，Loquat Leaf, Folium Eriobotryae］with its hair removed, Houpu［厚朴，Magnolia Bark, Cortex Magnoliae Officinalis］processed with ginger juice after its rough skin removed, 0.5 Liang of Dingxiang［丁香，Clove, Flos Caryophylli］, 1 Fen of Huoxiangye［藿香叶，Agastache leaf, Agastaches Folium］, 0.5 Liang of Gancao［甘草，Liquorice Root, Radix Glycyrrhizae］stir-fried, 0.5 Liang of Ganjiang［干姜，Dried Ginger, Rhizoma Zingiberis］processed, 0.5 Liang of Chenpi［陈皮，Dried Tangerine Peel, Pericarpium Citri Reticulatae］steeped in decoction after the pulp being removed.

上件一十二味，修事了，称分两，捣罗为末。每服二钱。水一大盏，入生姜钱一片，枣二枚，同煎至六分，去滓，温服。此药老人常服合吃。

Prepare and weigh all the above 12 kinds of medicinals as required, then pound them into powder. Take 2 Qian each time. Put it in a big cup of water, add a piece of fresh ginger as big as copper and 2 jujubes. Decoct until three fifths is left. Remove the residue and take it when it is warm. It is suitable for the aged to take regularly.

老人和脾胃气，治胸膈痞闷，心腹刺痛，不思饮食。枳壳木香散。男子女人通用此方。

Zhiqiao Muxiang San（Orange Fruit and Root of Common Aucklandia Powder）is used to regulate the spleen and stomach qi, treat chronic infectious disease, depression in the chest and diaphragm, stabbing pain in the heart and abdomen, and anorexia. It is suitable for both men and women generally.

木香一两　神曲杵末，炒，四两　荆三棱四两，炮　青橘皮去瓤，三两　甘草三两，炮　益智去皮，三两　白芷一两　桂心三两　莪术三两，炮　白术微炒，二两　枳壳麸炒，炮

The formula is composed of 1 Liang of Muxiang［木香, Root of Common Aucklandia, Radix Aucklandiae］, 4 Liang of Shenqu［神曲, Medicated Leaven, Massa Medicata Fermentata］pestled into powder and fried, 4 Liang of Jingsanleng［荆三棱, Scirpus, Scirpi Fluviatilis Rhizoma］processed, 3 Liang of Qingjupi［青橘皮, Unripe Tangerine Peel, Citri Reticulatae Pericarpium Viride］with the pulp removed, 3 Liang of Gancao［甘草, Liquorice Root, Radix Glycyrrhizae］processed, 3 Liang of Yizhi［益智, Sharp-leaf Glangal Fruit, Fructus Alpiniae Oxyphyllae］with the skin removed, 1 Liang of Baizhi［白芷, Root of Dahurian Angelica, Radix Angelicae Dahuricae］, 3 Liang of Guixin［桂心, Cinnamon Bark, Cortex Cinnamomi］, 3 Liang of Ezhu［莪术, Zedoray Rhizome, Rhizoma Curcumae］processed, 2 Liang of Baizhu［白术, Argehead Atractylodes Rhizome, Rhizoma Atractylodis Macrocephalae］fried slightly, Zhiqiao［枳壳, Orange Fruit, Fructus Aurantii］stir-fried with bran and processed.

上件药，捣罗为末。每服二钱，水一盏，入生姜、盐各少许，同煎至七分，并滓热服。

Pound the above medicinals into powder. Take 2 Qian each time. Put the powder in a cup of water, add a little fresh ginger and salt, decoct until seven tenths is left. Take the decoction together with dregs when it is warm.

解老人四时伤寒。四顺散。男子女人皆通用此方。

Sishun San（Four Regulation Powder）is used to treat cold damage of the aged in the four seasons, which is suitable for both men and women generally.

麻黄去节　杏仁去皮　甘草炙　荆芥穗以上各等分

It is composed of Mahuang［麻黄, Ephedra, Herba Ephedrae］with its nodes removed, Xingren［杏仁, Bitter Apricot Seed, Semen Armeniacae Amarum］with the skin removed, Gancao［甘草, Liquorice Root, Radix Glycyrrhizae］stir-fried, and Jingjiesui［荆芥穗, Schizonepeta Spike, Schizonepetae Flos］. Prepare the above medicinals in equal amount.

上同杵为末，每服一钱，入盐汤点热服。

Pound them into powder. Take 1 Qian each time. Swallow them with weak brine when it is hot.

治老人心脾积热，或流注，脚膝疼痛。黄芪散。男子女人通用。

Huangqi San（Astragalus Powder）can be used to treat accumulated heat in the heart and spleen, multiple abscess, pain in the feet and knees of the aged. It is suitable for both men and women generally.

黄芪　赤芍药　牡丹皮　香白芷　沙参　甘草炙　肉桂去皮　柴胡去苗　当归洗后炙

It is composed of Huangqi ［黄芪, Milkvetch Root, Radix Astragali seu Hedysari］, Chishaoyao ［赤芍药, Red Peony, Paeoniae Radix Rubra］, Mudanpi ［牡丹皮, Tree Peony Root Bark, Cortex Moutan Radicis］, Xiangbaizhi ［香白芷, Dahurian Angelica, Angelicae Dahuricae Radix］, Shashen ［沙参, Fourleaf Ladybell Root, Radix Adenophorae］, Gancao ［甘草, Liquorice Root, Radix Glycyrrhizae］ stir-fried, Rougui ［肉桂, Cassia Bark, Cortex Cinnamomi］ with the skin removed, Chaihu ［柴胡, Chinese thorowax root, Radix Bupleuri］ with the sprout removed, and Danggui ［当归, Chinese Angelica, Radix Angelicae Sinensis］ stir-fried after being washed.

上件等分，捣罗为末。每服二钱。水一盏，姜三片，煎至五分，日进三服。春冬每煎时，入蜜蒸瓜蒌煎半匙。忌粘食、炙煿等物。

Prepare the above medicinals in equal amount and pound them into powder. Take 2 Qian each time. Put 3 pieces of ginger into a cup of water. Decoct until half of it is left. Take it 3 times a day. When it is decocted in spring and winter, half spoon of Gualou ［瓜蒌, Trichosanthes, Trichosanthis

Fructus] steamed with honey can be added. It is contraindicated with the sticky or stir-fried food.

橘皮煮散。益元气，和脾胃，治伤寒。此名不换金散，但心腹诸疾，并用疗之。男子女人通用。

Jupizhusan (Powder of Tangerine Peel Decoction) is used to replenish original qi, harmonize the spleen and stomach, and treat cold damage. It is also called Invaluable Powder due to its great value. It can be used to treat all kinds of diseases related to the heart and abdomen. It is suitable for both men and women generally.

橘皮去瓤秤，一两用　人参　茯苓　白术各一两　木香一分　干姜炮　官桂半两，去皮称　槟榔一两，鸡心者用　草豆蔻二个，去皮　半夏一分，麸炒　厚朴半两，入姜一分同称，碎，炒干　枳壳半两，去瓤，麸炒　诃黎勒五个，煨熟去核　甘草半两

The formula is composed of 1 Liang of Jupi [橘皮, Tangerine Peel, Citri Reticulatae Pericarpium] weighed with the pulp removed, 1 Liang of Renshen [人参, Ginseng, Radix Ginseng], 1 Liang of Fuling [茯苓, Indian Bread, Poria], 1 Liang of Baizhu [白术, Argehead Atractylodes Rhizome, Rhizoma Atractylodis Macrocephalae], 1 Fen of Muxiang [木香, Root of Common Aucklandia, Radix Aucklandiae], Ganjiang [干姜, Dried Ginger, Rhizoma Zingiberis] processed, 0.5 Liang of Guangui [官桂, Cassia Cortex Cinnamomi] weighed with the skin removed, 1 Liang of Binglang [槟榔, Areca Seed, Semen Arecae] shaped like chicken heart, 2 Caodoukou [草豆蔻, Katsumada

Galangal Seed, Semen Alpiniae Katsumadai〕with the skin removed, 1 Fen of Banxia〔半夏, Pinellia Tuber, Rhizoma Pinelliae〕stir-fried with bran, 0.5 Liang of Houpu〔厚朴, Magnolia Bark, Cortex Magnoliae Officinalis〕and together with 1 Fen of ginger pounded into powder and stir-fried, 0.5 Liang of Zhiqiao〔枳壳, Orange Fruit, Fructus Aurantii〕stir-fried with bran after the pulp being removed, 5 Helile〔诃黎勒, Chebule, Chebulae Fructus〕stewed with their cores removed, and 0.5 Liang of Gancao〔甘草, Liquorice Root, Radix Glycyrrhizae〕.

上件，捣罗为末。每服一大钱，水一盏，姜枣同煎至七分，热吃。不问食前、食后并宜服，忌如常。

Pound the above ingredients into powder. Take 1 Qian each time. Put the powder, some ginger and Chinese dates in a cup of water and decoct until seven tenths is left. Take the decoction when it is hot. It can be taken before or after meals. The contraindication is as usual.

治老人脏腑冷热不调，里急后重，阑门不和。香白芷散。男子女人通用。

Xiangbaizhi San（Dahurian Angelica Powder）is used to treat irregularities of cold-heat in zang-fu organs, tenesmus, disorder of the intestines of the aged. It is suitable for both men and women generally.

当归三钱，洗　香白芷三钱，洗　茯苓三钱，去皮　枳壳三钱，麸炒　木香一钱

It is composed of 3 Qian of Danggui 〔当归, Chinese Angelica, Radix Angelicae Sinensis〕washed, 3 Qian of Xiangbaizhi 〔香白芷, Dahurian Angelica, Angelicae Dahuricae Radix〕washed, 3 Qian of Fuling 〔茯苓, Indian Bread, Poria〕with the skin removed, 3 Qian of Zhiqiao 〔枳壳, Orange Fruit, Fructus Aurantii〕stir-fried with bran, and 1 Qian of Muxiang 〔木香, Root of Common Aucklandia, Radix Aucklandiae〕.

上件为末。每服一钱,水半盏,生姜少许,同煎至四分,温服。

Pound the above ingredients into powder. Take 1 Qian each time. Put the powder and a little fresh ginger in a half cup of water and decoct until two fifths is left. Take the decoction when it is warm.

治老人大小便不通。匀气散。通用。

Yunqi San（Qi-Evening Powder）is used to treat constipation and urine retention of the aged. It is suitable for both men and women generally.

生姜半两　葱一茎,和根叶泥用　盐一捻　豉三十粒

It is composed of 0.5 Liang of Shengjiang 〔生姜, Fresh Ginger, Zingiberis Rhizoma Recens〕, a piece of Cong 〔葱, Scallion, Allium Fistulosum L.〕, a scallion with its root and leaves being mashed, a little salt, and 30 Douchi 〔豆豉, Fermented Soybean, Semen Sojae Preparatum〕.

上件四味捣烂,安脐中。良久,便通。

Pound the above 4 ingredients and put them in the navel. Wait for a fairly long time, the constipation and urine retention will be relieved.

治老人小便不通。地龙膏。

Dilong Gao（Earthworm Paste）is used to treat urine retention of the aged.

白项地龙，茴香用时看多少。

It is composed of Dilong［地龙, Earthworm, Pheretima］with white clitellum, and Huixiang［茴香, Fennel, Foeniculum Vulgare］, the amount of which depending on the real need.

上件杵汁，倾于脐内，自然便通。

Pestle the above ingredients into juice and pour it into the navel. Retention of urine will be cured naturally.

治老人脚膝疼痛，不能履地。七圣散。

Qisheng San（Powder of Seven Effective Medicinals）is used to treat pains in the knees and feet of the aged, and inability to walk.

杜仲一两　续断一两　萆薢一两　防风一两　独活一两　牛膝一两，酒浸一宿　甘草一两

It is composed of 1 Liang of Duzhong［杜仲, Eucommia Bark, Cortex Eucommiae］, 1 Liang of Xuduan［续断, Dipsacus, Dipsaci Radix］, 1 Liang of Bixie［萆薢, Rhizome of Hypoglaucous collett yam, Rhizoma Dioscoreae

Hypoglaucae〕, 1 Liang of Fangfeng〔防风, Divaricate Saposhnikovia Root, Radix Saposhnikoviae〕, 1 Liang of Duhuo〔独活, Pubescent Angelica, Radix Angelicae Pubescentis〕, 1 Liang of Niuxi〔牛膝, Twotoothed Achyranthes Root, Radix Achyranthis Bidentatae〕steeped in liquor for a night, and 1 Liang of Gancao〔甘草, Liquorice Root, Radix Glycyrrhizae〕.

上件为末。每服二钱，酒调下。

Pound the above ingredients into powder. Take 2 Qian with liquor each time.

治老人脾胃一切病。温白丸。兼治脾不承受，吐逆、泻痢，及宿食不消方。通用。

Wenbai Wan (White Atractylodes Pill with Warming Function) is used to treat all diseases about the spleen and stomach of the aged. It is also effective to treat vomiting, diarrhea and retained food due to the disorder of the spleen. It is suitable for all people.

半夏二两，汤洗，姜汁浸　白术一两，炮　丁香一分

It is composed of 2 Liang of Banxia〔半夏, Pinellia Tuber, Rhizoma Pinelliae〕washed with decoction and steeped in ginger juice, 1 Liang of Baizhu〔白术, Argehead Atractylodes Rhizome, Rhizoma Atractylodis Macrocephalae〕processed, and 1 Fen of Dingxiang〔丁香, Clove, Flos Caryophylli〕.

上件为末，用生姜自然汁，和飞面为糊，捣和前药末为丸，如梧桐子大。浓煎生姜汤下十丸，空心服。如腹疼并呕逆，食后。

Pound the above ingredients into powder. Mix fresh ginger juice with fine flour into paste. Pound the powder and the paste into pills as big as firmiana seeds. Decoct fresh ginger juice to a thick state and take 10 pills with it on an empty stomach. If there is stomach ache, vomiting and counter-flow, take it after meals.

藁本散。治妇人血气，丈夫筋骨风，四肢软弱，及卒中急风，并寸白虫，但常服并皆攻治。或要出汗，解伤寒，汤使如后。此方是孟相公进过。

Gaoben San (Chinese Lovage Powder) is used to treat menstrual irregularities of woman, pains in sinews and bones of man, weak limbs, hemiplegia and facial distortion due to stroke, and eliminate tapeworms. The long-term taking of it will cure all those diseases. If it is used to promote sweating and relieve cold damage, the guiding drugs listed below can be referred. This formula was ever used by the prime minister named Meng.

藁本　牛膝酒浸一宿，焙干　当归　麻黄去节。以上各一两　羌活　独活　防风　肉桂去粗皮秤　芍药　菊花以上各半两　续断　五加皮　芎䓖　甘草　赤箭　枳壳麸炒，去瓤。以上各半两　黑附子大者一个，炮去皮脐　细辛一分，去叶秤

It is composed of 1 Liang of Gaoben [藁本, Chinese Lovage, Ligustici Rhizoma], 1 Liang of Niuxi [牛膝, Twotoothed Achyranthes Root, Radix

Achyranthis Bidentatae〕dried after steeped in liquor for a night, 1 Liang of Danggui〔当归, Chinese Angelica, Radix Angelicae Sinensis〕, 1 Liang of Mahuang〔麻黄, Ephedra, Herba Ephedrae〕with its nodes removed, 0.5 Liang of Qianghuo〔羌活, Incised Notopterygium Rhizome and Root, Rhizoma et Radix Notopterygii〕, 0.5 Liang of Duhuo〔独活, Pubescent Angelica, Radix Angelicae Pubescentis〕, 0.5 Liang of Fangfeng〔防风, Divaricate Saposhnikovia Root, Radix Saposhnikoviae〕, 0.5 Liang of Rougui〔肉桂, Cassia Bark, Cortex Cinnamomi〕weighed with the rough skin removed, 0.5 Liang of Shaoyao〔芍药, Chinese Herbaceous Peony, Paeonia lactiflora Pall.〕, 0.5 Liang of Juhua〔菊花, Chrysanthemums, Dendranthema Morifolium Tzvel.〕, 0.5 Liang of Xuduan〔续断, Dipsacus, Dipsaci Radix〕, 0.5 Liang of Wujiapi〔五加皮, Slenderstyle Acanthopanax Bark, Cortex Acanthopanax Radicis〕, 0.5 Liang of Xiongqiong〔芎䓖, Sichuan Lovage Rhizome, Rhizoma Ligustici Chuanxiong〕, 0.5 Liang of Gancao〔甘草, Liquorice Root, Radix Glycyrrhizae〕, 0.5 Liang of Chijian〔赤箭, Rhizome of Tall Gastrodia, Rhizoma Gastrodiae〕, 0.5 Liang of Zhiqiao〔枳壳, Orange Fruit, Fructus Aurantii〕stir-fried with bran after the pulp being removed, a big black Fuzi〔附子, Sliced Aconite, Aconiti Radix Lateralis Denigrata〕processed with the skin and navel removed, and 1 Fen of Xixin〔细辛, Asarum, Asarum sieboldii Miq.〕weighed with the leaves removed.

上件药一十八味,并须州土好者。使水洗过,细锉,焙干,捣罗为末。空心,温酒下二钱。如不饮酒,薄荷汤下。发汗,解伤寒热,葱白酒下二钱,并服三五服为妙。

Collect the above 18 kinds of medicinals from the region noted for the drugs. Wash, file, dry them and pound them into powder. Take 2 Qian of the powder with warm liquor on an empty stomach. Peppermint decoction can be a substitute for people who do not drink wine. Take 2 Qian together with scallion and liquor and have it for 3 to 5 doses, which is effective to induce sweating and treat fever caused by cold damage.

治老人风冷，展筋骨。续断散方。

Xuduan San（Dipsacus Powder）is used to treat spasm and severe pain due to wind cold, and regulate sinews and bones of the aged.

续断一两　牛膝二两　川芎一两　木瓜二两

It is composed of 1 Liang of Xuduan［续断, Dipsacus, Dipsaci Radix］, 2 Liang of Niuxi［牛膝, Twotoothed Achyranthes Root, Radix Achyranthis Bidentatae］, 1 Liang of Chuanxiong［川芎, Sichuan Lovage Rhizome, Ligusticum chuanxiong Hort.］, and 2 Liang of Mugua［木瓜, Common Floweringqince Fruit, Fructus Chaenomelis］.

上为细末。空心时，温酒调下一大钱。

Pound the above ingredients into fine powder. Take 1 Qian of it with warm liquor on an empty stomach.

坠痰化涎，和脾胃。人参半夏丸。

Renshen Banxia Wan（Ginseng and Pinellia Pill）is used to transform phlegm and saliva, and harmonize the spleen and stomach.

半夏一两　生姜四两，取汁，先以汤洗半夏七遍，浸三日后，于日内煎干，切作饼子，焙干　白矾一两　人参一两　茯苓一两，去皮

It is composed of 1 Liang of Banxia〔半夏，Pinellia Tuber, Rhizoma Pinelliae〕, 4 Liang of Shengjiang〔生姜，Fresh Ginger, Zingiberis Rhizoma Recens〕with the juice preserved. Wash Banxia in the juice for 7 times, steep it for 3 days, stir-fry it in one day, cut it into pancakes and dry it. Prepare 1 Liang of Baifan〔白矾，alum, Alumen〕, 1 Liang of Renshen〔人参，ginseng, Radix Ginseng〕, and 1 Liang of Fuling〔茯苓，Indian Bread, Poria〕with the skin removed.

上为末，以蒸饼水浸过，却用纸裹，煨熟为丸，如绿豆大。每日空心，夜卧，用淡生姜汤下十五丸。开胃口，姜枣汤下。风涎，用皂角一条，姜三片，萝卜三片，同煎汤下。

Pound the above ingredients into powder. Steep the powder in water that has steamed the pancakes. Wrap it with paper. Roast it and then make it into pills as big as mung beans. Take it on an empty stomach each day. Swallow 15 pills with light fresh ginger decoction when going to bed. If taking with ginger and jujube decoction, the appetite can be stimulated. If taking with decoction made of one bar of Zaojiao〔皂角，gleditsia, Gleditsiae Fructus〕, 3 pieces of ginger and 3 pieces of turnip, wind-salvation can be treated.

治老人，暖食药。丁香丸。消食，治一切气闷，止醋心，腹胀，利胸膈，

逐积滞方。男子妇人通用。

Dingxiang Wan（Clove Pill）is a kind of stomach warming medicinals for the aged. It can be used to promote digestion, treat all kinds of labored breathing, stop acid regurgitation, treat abdominal distention, disinhibit chest and diaphragm, and expel stagnation. It is suitable for both men and women generally.

大乌梅一个，须是有裙襕者　巴豆一个，新肥者和皮用　香墨末炒，半钱　拣丁香五个，须是新者用　胡椒五粒，须是黑者　干漆末炒，半钱，先炒为末　桂花末炒，半钱，香墨、干漆、桂花三味研入

It is composed of one big Wumei［乌梅, Smoked Plum, Fructus Mume］with rich pulp, one Badou［巴豆, Croton Fruit, Fructus Crotonis］chosen from the new and round ones and used with its skin unremoved, 0.5 Qian of Xiangmo［香墨, Ink, Atramentum］stir-fried to powder. Select 5 new Dingxiang［丁香, Clove, Flos Caryophylli］, and 5 grains of black Hujiao［胡椒, Pepper, Piperis Fructus］. Prepare 0.5 Qian of Ganqi［干漆, Dried Lacquer, Resina Toxicodendri］stir-fried to powder, 0.5 Qian of the powder of Guihua［桂花, Murraya Jasminorage, Folium et Cacumen Murrayae］stir-fried. Grind the above 3 ingredients of Xiangmo, Ganqi and Guihua.

上为末，用马尾罗子罗过，用醋面糊为剂，臼中杵令匀，如绿豆大。温酒下五丸至七丸，茶下亦得。或入蜡茶末炒三钱更妙。

Pound the above ingredients into powder. Filter them with sieve. Then put the filtered fine powder and vinegar into flour to make paste. Pestle the paste into smaller pills as big as mung beans. Swallow 5 to 7 pills with warm liquor or tea. It would be better to stir-fry to powder with 3 Qian of wax tea.

香草散。治妇人气羸，肠寒便白，食伤积滞，冷结肠不成。温脾肺，活荣生肌，进食，益冲任二经。

Xiangcao San（Musk Herb Powder）is used to treat qi deficiency of women, coldness of the intestines, disorder of stool, and cold stagnation due to food accumulation. It is also used to warm the spleen and the lung, nourish the nutrient qi, promote tissue regeneration, stimulate appetite, and benefit the thoroughfare and conception vessels.

茼茹　桔梗　白芷　当归　地榆　芍药　槟榔　白豆蔻各半两　麝香一钱

It is composed of 0.5 Liang of Lüru［茼茹, Lanru Herb, Herba Lanru］, 0.5 Liang of Jiegeng［桔梗, Platycodon Root, Platycodon grandiflorus A. DC.］, 0.5 Liang of Baizhi［白芷, Root of Dahurian Angelica, Radix Angelicae Dahuricae］, 0.5 Liang of Danggui［当归, Chinese Angelica, Radix Angelicae Sinensis］, 0.5 Liang of Diyu［地榆, Garden Burnet Root, Radix Sanguisorbae］, 0.5 Liang of Shaoyao［芍药, Chinese Herbaceous Peony, Paeonia lactiflora Pall］, 0.5 Liang of Binglang［槟榔, Areca Seed, Semen Arecae］, 0.5 Liang of Baidoukou［白豆蔻, Cardamon Fruit, Fructus Ammomi Rotundus］, and 1 Qian of Shexiang［麝香, Musk, Moschus］.

上为末。每服二钱，水一盏，姜枣同煎，至数沸，通口，食前，日进三分。

Pound the above ingredients into powder. Put 2 Qian of the powder along with ginger and jujubes into a cup of water. Decoct them to the boiling state. Take it before meal and 3 times a day.

香枳汤。治老人大肠秘涩。调风顺气。男子妇人通用。

Xiangzhi Tang (Bitter Orange Decoction) is used to treat constipation of the aged. It can remove wind pathogen and regulate the qi flow of the body. It is suitable for both men and women generally.

枳壳去瓤，麸炒　防风一两　甘草半两，炙

It is composed of Zhiqiao [枳壳, Orange Fruit, Fructus Aurantii] stir-fried with bran after the pulp being removed, 1 Liang of Fangfeng [防风, Divaricate Saposhnikovia Root, Radix Saposhnikoviae], and 0.5 Liang of Gancao [甘草, Liquorice Root, Radix Glycyrrhizae] stir-fried.

上为末。每服二钱，百沸汤点服。空心、食前各一服。

Pound the above ingredients into powder. Take 2 Qian of it each time with boiling soup. Take one dose each on an empty stomach and before meal.

治妇人男子久积虚败。壮元补血，健胃暖脾，止痰逆，消饮食。北亭丸。

Beiting Wan (Sal Ammoniac Pill) is used to treat abdominal mass and emaciation of women and men. It is effective to supplement original qi and tonify blood, invigorate the stomach, warm the spleen, remove phlegm, stop counterflow of qi, and promote digestion.

北亭砂二两，去除砂石　阿魏半两，同硇砂研令细，醋化，去砂石　川当归净洗，去苗稍用　厚朴去皮，姜汁炙，令黄色　陈橘皮去瓤用红　官桂去皮秤　干姜炮　甘草炙　川芎　胡椒拣好者　缩砂去皮用　大附子炮，去皮脐。以上各秤四两　茯苓二两　青盐二两，与硇砂、阿魏同醋研，去沙土　白术米泔水浸一宿，切作片子，焙干　五味子一两半，去沙土用之

It is composed of 2 Liang of Beitingsha ［北亭砂, Sal Ammoniac, Sal Ammoniac］ with the sand removed, 0.5 Liang of Awei ［阿魏, Chinese Asafetida, Resina Ferulae］ pounded together with Naosha ［硇砂, Sal Ammoniac, Sal Ammoniacum］ acetified with the sand removed, 4 Liang of Chuandanggui ［川当归, Sichuan Tangkuei, Angelicae Sinensis Radix］ washed with the sprout removed, 4 Liang of Houpu ［厚朴, Magnolia Bark, Cortex Magnoliae Officinalis］ with the skin removed and ginger juice stir-fried to brown, 4 Liang of Chenjupi ［陈橘皮, Dried Tangerine Peel, Pericarpium Citri Reticulatae］ with the pulp removed, 4 Liang of Guangui ［官桂, Cassia Cortex Cinnamomi］ weighed with the skin removed, 4 Liang of Ganjiang ［干姜, Dried Ginger, Rhizoma Zingiberis］ processed, 4 Liang of Gancao ［甘草, Liquorice Root, Radix Glycyrrhizae］ stir-fried, 4 Liang of Chuanxiong ［川芎, Sichuan Lovage Rhizome, Ligusticum chuanxiong Hort.］, 4 Liang of fine Hujiao ［胡椒, Pepper, Piperis Fructus］, 4 Liang of Suosha ［缩砂, Fructus Amomi Xanthioidis, Amomum villosum Lour. Var.xanthioides T.L.Wu et Senjen］ with the skin removed, 4 Liang of big Fuzi ［附子, Aconite, Radix Aconiti Praeparata］ processed with the skin and navel removed, 2 Liang of

Fuling［茯苓, Indian Bread, Poria］, 2 Liang of Qingyan［青盐, Halite, Halitum］ processed with vinegar together with Naosha and Awei with the sand removed, Baizhu［白术, Argehead Atractylodes Rhizome, Rhizoma Atractylodis Macrocephalae］ steeped in rice water for a night and sliced then dried, and 1.5 Liang of Wuweizi［五味子, Chinese Magnoliavine Fruit, Fructus Schisandrae Chinensis］ with the sand removed.

上件，依法修事为末。将硇砂、阿魏、醋入面，看多少同煎稀糊，下药。更炼好蜜，同搜和拌匀，再入臼中杵千百下，丸如酸枣大。每服一丸，空心，盐汤茶酒任下，嚼破。妇人一切病患，并宜服此。

Process the above ingredients into powder. Put Naosha, Awei and vinegar into flour and make them into paste. Put the powder in the paste. It would be better to add refined honey and then pestle the mixture thousands of times in a mortar. Make it into pills as big as spine date. Take one pill each time on an empty stomach. Chew and swallow it with brine, tea or wine. It is useful to treat all kinds of female diseases.

治老人一切风。乌犀丸。

Wuxi Wan（Gleditschia Horrida Pill）is used to treat wind diseases of the aged.

天麻二两　地榆一两　元参一两　川乌头一两, 炮制去皮　龙脑薄荷四两　藿香叶一两　皂角三挺, 不蛀者, 烧红, 入水中浸之　龙脑少许　麝香少许

It is composed of 2 Liang of Tianma［天麻, Tall Gastrodia, Gastrodiae

Rhizoma], 1 Liang of Diyu [地榆, Garden Burnet Root, Radix Sanguisorbae], 1 Liang of Yuanshen [元参, Root of Ningpo Figwort, Radix Scrophulariae], 1 Liang of Chuanwutou [川乌头, Radix Aconiti Sinensis, Aconiti Radix] processed with the skin removed, 4 Liang of Longnaobohe [龙脑薄荷, Baikal Betony Herb, Herba Stachydis Baicalensis], 1 Liang of Huoxiangye [藿香叶, Agastache Leaf, Agastaches Folium], 3 fine Zaojiao [皂角, Gleditsia, Gleditsiae Fructus] first baked and then steeped in water, a little Longnao [龙脑, Borneol, Borneolum], and a little Shexiang [麝香, Musk, Moschus].

上为末，炼蜜为膏，如皂子大。每服一丸，嚼吃。小儿半丸以下。薄荷、茶、酒调下。

Pound the above ingredients into powder. Process it with honey into pills as big as gleditsia seed. Chew one pill each time. Less than half a pill is suitable for children. Take it with Bohe [薄荷, Peppermint, Herba Menthae], tea, or liquor.

镇心丸。养老人心气，令不健忘，聪耳明目方。

Zhenxin Wan (Heart-Settling Pill) is used to nourish the heart qi of the old, prevent amnesia, and improve hearing and vision.

辰砂一两　桂一两　远志去心　人参以上各一两　茯苓二两　麦门冬去心　石菖蒲　干地黄各一两半　以上除辰砂，并为末，合匀

It is composed of 1 Liang of Chensha [辰砂, Cinnabar, Vermilion Mercuric Blende], 1 Liang of Gui [桂, Cassia Twig, Ramulus Cinnamomi], 1 Liang of

Yuanzhi［远志, Polygala Root, Radix Polygalae］with the pith discarded, 1 Liang of Renshen［人参, Ginseng, Radix Ginseng］, 2 Liang of Fuling［茯苓, Indian Bread, Poria］, 1.5 Liang of Maimendong［麦门冬, Radix Ophiopogonis, Ophiopogon japonicus Ker-Gawl］with the pith discarded, 1.5 Liang of Shichangpu［石菖蒲, Grassleaf Sweetflag Rhizome, Rhizoma Acori Tatarinowii］, and 1.5 Liang of dried Dihuang［地黄, Rehmannia, Radix Rehmanniae］. Pound the above ingredients except Chensha into powder and mix them well.

上，炼蜜为末，丸如桐子大。空心，薄荷酒吞下十丸至十五丸。留少朱砂为衣，益心气养神，宜常服。

Process the powder with honey into pills as big as firmiana seeds. Swallow down 10 to 15 pills with peppermint wine on an empty stomach. Smaller amount of Zhusha［朱砂, Cinnabar, Cinnabaris］can be kept to avoid damage of the liver and kidney, and to replenish the heart qi and spirit. It is suitable to take regularly.

治老人脾肺客热，上焦滞痰。凉心、润肺、消壅。枇杷叶散。男子女人通用。

Pipaye San（Loquat Leaf Powder）is used to treat invading fever in the spleen and the lung of the aged, stagnation of phlegm in the upper energizer, clear heart heat, moisten the lung, and expel stagnation. It is suitable for both men and women generally.

枇杷叶炙，去毛　人参　茯苓　白术　羌活　黄芪一两　甘草炙　半夏汤洗去滑，切破焙干，各半两

The formula is composed of 1 Liang of Pipaye［枇杷叶, Loquat Leaf, Folium Eriobotryae］stir-fried with its hair removed, 1 Liang of Renshen［人参, Ginseng, Radix Ginseng］, 1 Liang of Fuling［茯苓, Indian Bread, Poria］, 1 Liang of Baizhu［白术, Argehead Atractylodes Rhizome, Rhizoma Atractylodis Macrocephalae］, 1 Liang of Qianghuo［羌活, Incised Notopterygium Rhizome and Root, Rhizoma et Radix Notopterygii］, 1 Liang of Huangqi［黄芪, Milkvetch Root, Radix Astragali seu Hedysari］, 0.5 Liang of Gancao［甘草, Liquorice Root, Radix Glycyrrhizae］stir-fried, and 0.5 Liang of Banxia［半夏, Pinellia Tuber, Rhizoma Pinelliae］cut and dried after its serous fluid being removed by washing.

上为末。每服二钱，水一盏，入生姜、薄荷，煎至七分，食后、临卧温服。

Pound the above ingredients into powder. Take 2 Qian each time. Put the powder, fresh ginger and Bohe［薄荷, Peppermint, Herba Menthae］into a cup of water and decoct until seven tenths left. Take the decoction when it is warm after dinner and before going to sleep.

羌活散。治老人耳聋眼暗，头项腰背疼痛，浑身疮癣，此乃肾脏风所攻也。

Qianghuo San（Incised Notopterygium Rhizome and Root Powder）is used to treat deafness and blurred vision, pains in the head, neck and back, sores and tinea on the body of the aged, which are caused by the wind-dampness attacking the kidney.

羌活　枳壳麸炒去瓤　半夏汤浸七遍　甘草炙　大腹子　防风　桑白皮各等分

The formula is composed of Qianghuo ［羌活, Incised Notopterygium Rhizome and Root, Rhizoma et Radix Notopterygii］, Zhiqiao ［枳壳, Orange Fruit, Fructus Aurantii］ stir-fried with bran after the pulp is removed, Banxia ［半夏, Pinellia Tuber, Rhizoma Pinelliae］ steeped in decoction for 7 times, Gancao ［甘草, Liquorice Root, Radix Glycyrrhizae］ stir-fried, Dafuzi ［大腹子, Areca, Arecae Semen］, Fangfeng ［防风, Divaricate Saposhnikovia Root, Radix Saposhnikoviae］ and Sangbaipi ［桑白皮, White Mulberry Root-bark, Cortex Mori］ in equal amount.

上为粗末。每服二钱，水一盏，生姜煎至七分，温服。早辰、日午时，临卧各一服。

Pound the above ingredients into crude powder. Take 2 Qian each time. Put the powder and fresh ginger in a cup of water and decoct until seven tenths is left. Take one dose when it is warm in the morning, at noon and in the evening before sleep respectively.

搜风顺气，治老人百疾。七圣丸。男子女人通用。

Qisheng Wan（Pill of Seven Effective Medicinals）is used to track wind pathogen and guide qi downward, and treat all kinds of wind diseases of the aged. It is suitable for both men and women generally.

槟榔　木香一两　川芎　羌活　桂心各一两　郁李仁一两，去皮尖，炒令黄色　大黄一两一分，炒

It is composed of 1 Liang of Binglang［槟榔, Areca Seed, Semen Arecae］, 1 Liang of Muxiang［木香, Root of Common Aucklandia, Radix Aucklandiae］, 1 Liang of Chuanxiong［川芎, Sichuan Lovage Rhizome, Ligusticum chuanxiong Hort.］, 1 Liang of Qianghuo［羌活, Incised Notopterygium Rhizome and Root, Rhizoma et Radix Notopterygii］, 1 Liang of Guixin［桂心, Cinnamon Bark, Cortex Cinnamomi］, 1 Liang of Yuliren［郁李仁, Chinese Dwarf Cherry Seed, Semen Pruni］ with the skin and pith removed and then stir-fried to brown, and 1.1 Liang of Dahuang［大黄, Rhubarb, Radix et Rhizoma Rhei］ stir-fried.

上为末，炼蜜为丸，桐子大。不计时候，温酒下七丸。要利动，即加七丸。淡姜汤下亦得。

Pound the above ingredients into powder. Process it with honey into pills as big as firmiana seeds. It can be taken anytime. Swallow 7 pills each time with warm wine. To achieve quick effect, 7 more pills can be taken and swallowed with light ginger decoction.

春时摄养第九

Chapter 9　Health Preservation in Spring

春属木，主发生。宜戒杀，茂于恩惠，以顺生气。春，肝气旺，肝属木，其味酸，木能胜土。土属脾主甘，当春之时，其饮食之味，宜减酸益甘以养脾气。肝气之盛者，调虚气以利之。顺之则安，逆之则少阳不生，肝气内变。

Spring pertains to the wood, representing the beginning of generation. It is advisable to quit killing, to let myriads of things prosper, and to adapt to the generating qi. In spring, liver qi is prosperous. The liver corresponds to the wood, and it is sour in taste. Wood restricts earth. The earth corresponds to the spleen and governs the sweetness. In spring, the aged should take less sour and more sweet in taste to nourish the spleen qi. For those who are exuberant in liver qi, exhale slowly to benefit it. If following the law, one will be healthy. If going against it, the Shaoyang（one kind of meridian in TCM）will not bring its function into full play, and the function of the liver will become abnormal.

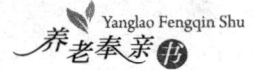

春时阳气初升，万物萌发，正二月间，乍寒乍热。高年之人，多有宿疾，春气所攻，则精神昏倦，宿患发动。又复经冬已来，拥炉熏衾，啗炙饮热，至春成积，多所发泄。致体热头昏，膈壅涎嗽，四肢劳倦，腰脚不任，皆冬所发之疾也，常宜体候。若稍利，恐伤脏腑。别生和气，凉膈化痰之药消解；或只选食治方中性稍凉、利饮食，调停与进，自然通畅。

In spring, the yang qi rises and everything germinates. In the second lunar month, it is alternatively cold and hot. The aged tend to be attacked by pathogenic factors in spring and suffer from somnolence. In this case, their abiding ailment is easy to be induced. In addition, in the winter that has just been over, the aged often sit around the stove with warm clothes, eat roasted meat and drink hot soup. It is not until the spring that all the accumulated heat may be vented. The following symptoms are all related to winter diseases such as fever, dizziness, stagnation in the diaphragm caused by salivation and coughing, fatigue of the limbs, and inflexibility of waist and feet. Therefore, it is suggested to understand and differentiate these syndromes well. To relieve constipation and urine retention with purging method may damage the zang-fu organs. Only the mild medicinal can be chosen as the treatment for the aged, differing from the traditional way for the common people. Diaphragm cooling and phlegm transforming medicinals can be used to resolve the internal and external pathogenic factors. Food that is neutral and slightly cool in diet therapy can also be chosen, which helps increase appetite. If the diet is regulated and taken properly, the diseases will be naturally cured.

若别无疾状，不须服药，常择和暖日，引侍尊亲于园亭楼阁虚敞之处，使放意登眺，用摅滞怀，以畅生气。时寻花木游赏，以快其意，不令孤坐独眠，自生郁闷；春时若亲朋请召，老人意欲从欢，任自遨游。常令嫡亲侍从，惟酒不可过饮；春时人家多造冷馔、米食等，不令下与；如水团兼粽、粘冷肥僻之物，多伤脾胃，难得消化，大不益老人，切宜看承。春时遇天气燠暖，不可顿减绵衣。缘老人气弱、骨疏怯，风冷易伤肌体。但多穿夹衣，遇暖之时，一重渐减一重，即不致暴伤也。今具春时汤药如后。

There is no need to take medicine if no other symptoms occur. When it is warm, guide and accompany the aged to the spacious places outdoors such as beautiful gardens or pavilions. Let them enjoy a distant view to get rid of unpleasant things and free the vital qi. Let them enjoy beautiful flowers and trees now and then to make the aged happy. Do not let them sit and sleep alone to avoid depression. In spring, if relatives and friends invite the aged to their home, let them feel free to go and enjoy themselves to the full. Make sure they are accompanied and not drunk during the process. In spring, people often make more cold food, rice diet, etc., so do not let the aged accept such kind of food like rice dumplings, sticky, cold and fat things. These things, being harmful to the aged, are hard to digest and can damage the spleen and stomach, so the aged should be attended carefully to avoid improper food. Even it is warm in spring, the aged can not take off their thick clothes immediately because they are weak in essential qi and physique, and are susceptible to wind-cold. By wearing more thick clothes and taking off one item each time gradually when it is warm, the aged will not be seriously damaged suddenly. The formulas can be used in spring are listed below.

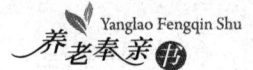

春时用诸药方
Formulas for the Aged in Spring

治老人春时多昏倦。细辛散。明目，和脾胃，除风气，去痰涎。男子女人通用。

Xixin San (Asarum Powder) can be used to treat somnolence of the aged in spring. It improves vision, harmonizes the spleen and stomach, removes wind pathogen and disperses phlegm and saliva. It is suitable for both men and women generally.

细辛一两，去土　川芎二两　甘草半两，炙

It is composed of 1 Liang of Xixin [细辛, Asarum, Asarum sieboldii Miq.] with the earth removed, 2 Liang of Chuanxiong [川芎, Sichuan Lovage Rhizome, Rhizoma Ligustici Chuanxiong], and 0.5 Liang of Gancao [甘草, Liquorice Root, Radix Glycyrrhizae] stir-fried.

上为末。每服一大钱，一水一盏，煎至六分，热呷。可常服。

Pound the above ingredients into powder. Take 1 Qian each time. Put the powder into a cup of water and decoct until three fifths is left. Sip the decoction when it is hot. It can be taken regularly.

治老人春时热毒，风攻颈项，头痛面肿，及风毒眼涩。菊花散。

Juhua San (Chrysanthemum Powder) can be used to remove heat toxin of the aged in spring, to treat stiff neck attacked by the wind, headache and swollen face, and dry eyes due to wind toxin.

菊花　前胡　旋覆花　芍药　元参　苦参　防风各等分

It is composed of the following medicinals in equal amount: Juhua［菊花, Chrysanthemums, Dendranthema Morifolium Tzvel.］, Qianhu［前胡, radix peucedani, Peucedanum praeruptorum Dunn］, Xuanfuhua［旋覆花, Inula Flower, Flos Inula Japonica］, Shaoyao［芍药, Chinese Herbaceous Peony, Paeonia lactiflora Pall］, Yuanshen［元参, Root of Ningpo Figwort, Radix Scrophulariae］, Kushen［苦参, Lightyellow Sophora Root, Radix Sophorae Flavescentis］, and Fangfeng［防风, Divaricate Saposhnikovia Root, Radix Saposhnikoviae］.

上为末。食后临卧，用温酒调下三钱。不饮酒，用米饮调下亦得。

Pound the above ingredients into powder. Take 3 Qian of it with warm liquor after dinner and before sleeping. Rice beverage can be a substitute for the liquor.

治老人春时头目不利，昏昏如醉，壮热头疼，有似伤寒。惺惺丸。通用。

Xingxing Wan（Clever Pill）is used to treat disorders of the head and eyes of the aged in spring, including dizziness, high fever and headache, and symptoms like cold damage. It is suitable for both men and women generally.

桔梗　细辛　人参　甘草　茯苓　瓜蒌根　白术各一两

It is composed of 1 Liang of Jiegeng ［桔梗, Platycodon Root, Platycodon grandiflorus A. DC.］, 1 Liang of Xixin ［细辛, Asarum, Asarum sieboldii Miq.］, 1 Liang of Renshen ［人参, Ginseng, Radix Ginseng］, 1 Liang of Gancao ［甘草, Liquorice Root, Radix Glycyrrhizae］, 1 Liang of Fuling ［茯苓, Indian Bread, Poria］, 1 Liang of Gualougen ［瓜蒌根, Trichosanthes Root, Trichosanthis Radix］, and 1 Liang of Baizhu ［白术, Argehead Atractylodes Rhizome, Rhizoma Atractylodis Macrocephalae］.

上为末，炼蜜为丸，如弹子大，每服一丸，温水化破。治头痛腰痛，药入口，当下便惺惺。

Pound the above ingredients into powder. Process it with honey into pills as big as marbles. Take one pill each time and dissolve it in warm water. It can be used to treat headache and lumbago. As long as it is taken, the patient will feel better.

治老人春时多偏正头疼。神效方。通用。

Shenxiao Fang（Wondrous Effect Formula）is a very effective formula to treat medial headache and migraine of the aged in spring. It is suitable for both men and women generally.

旋覆花一两，焙　白僵蚕一两，炒　石膏一分，细研

It is composed of 1 Liang of Xuanfuhua ［旋覆花, Inula Flower, Flos Inula Japonica］ baked, 1 Liang of fried Baijiangcan ［白僵蚕, Silkworm

Larva, Larva Bombycis], and 1 Fen of ground Shigao [石膏, Gypsum, Gypsum Fibrosum].

上件为末,以葱煨熟,和根同杵为丸桐子大。急痛,用葱、茶下二丸。慢痛,不过二服。

Pound the above ingredients into powder. Roast it with scallion till it is cooked. Mix it with root and pestle it into pills as big as firmiana seeds. If there is a sharp pain, 2 pills can be taken with scallion and tea. If there is a chronic pain, 2 doses of it will work.

治老人春时胸膈不利,或时满闷。坠痰饮子。

Zhuitan Yinzi (Downbear Phlegm Decoction) is used to treat inhibited chest and diaphragm, or occasional vexation and oppression of the aged in spring.

半夏不计多少,用汤水洗十遍,为末　生姜一大块　枣七枚

It is composed of Banxia [半夏, Pinellia Tuber, Rhizoma Pinelliae] washed by hot water for 10 times and then pounded into powder, 1 big chunk of Shengjiang [生姜, Fresh Ginger, Zingiberis Rhizoma Recens] and 7 Zao [枣, jujube, Jujubae Fructus]

上二味,以水二盏,药末二钱,慢火煎至七分,临卧时,去生姜频服。

Put the above 2 medicinals with 2 Qian of Pinellia Tuber Powder into 2 cups of water. Decoct until seven tenths is left. Take it frequently when going to bed with the ginger removed.

老人春时，宜吃延年草，进食顺气，御药院常合进。通用。

Yannian Cao (Lifespan-Prolonging Powder) is used to promote appetite and regulate qi of the aged in spring. It is often used by imperial pharmacy. It is suitable for men and women generally.

青橘皮四两，浸洗，去瓤　甘草二两，为细末　盐二两半，炒

It is composed of 4 Liang of Qingjupi [青橘皮, Unripe Tangerine Peel, Citri Reticulatae Pericarpium Viride] steeped in decoction with the pulp removed, 2 Liang of Gancao [甘草, Liquorice Root, Radix Glycyrrhizae] ground into fine powder, and 2.5 Liang of salt that is fried.

上三味，先洗浸橘皮，去苦水，微焙，入甘草同焙干，后入盐，每早晨，嚼三两叶子，通滞气大好。

For the 3 medicinals, wash and steep the Qingjupi first, remove the bitter taste, then bake it slightly. Add Gancao and dry them, and then add the salt. Every morning, chew 3 or 2 pieces, which is useful to activate the stagnated qi.

治老人春时，诸般眼疾发动。黄芪散。兼治口鼻生疮。

Huangqi San (Astragalus Powder) is used to treat various eye diseases of the aged in spring. It can also be used to treat mouth and nose sores.

黄芪　川芎　防风　甘草　白蒺藜略炒，杵去尖，出火毒。以上各一两
甘菊花三分，不得用新菊

The formula is composed of 1 Liang of Huangqi 〔黄芪，Milkvetch Root, Radix Astragali seu Hedysari〕, 1 Liang of Chuanxiong 〔川芎，Sichuan Lovage Rhizome, Ligusticum chuanxiong Hort.〕, 1 Liang of Fangfeng 〔防风，Divaricate Saposhnikovia Root, Radix Saposhnikoviae〕, 1 Liang of Gancao〔甘草, Liquorice Root, Radix Glycyrrhizae〕, 1 Liang of Baijili〔白蒺藜，Puncturevine Caltrop Fruit, Fructus Tribuli〕fried slightly with the pith and heat toxin removed through pounding, and 3 Fen of Ganjuhua 〔甘菊花，Chrysanthemum, Chrysanthemi Flos〕but not new chrysanthemum.

上，净洗晒干，勿更近火，捣为末。每服二钱，早晨空心、日午、临卧各一服，干咽或米饮调下。暴赤风毒，泪昏涩痛痒等眼，只三服，三两日永效。内外障眼，久服方退。忌房室、毒物、火上食。凡患眼，切不得头上针络出血，及服皂角、牵牛等药，取一时之快，并大损眼。

Wash the above ingredients and dry them. Leave them away from the fire. Then pound them into powder. Take 2 Qian each time and 3 times a day. Take it in the morning on an empty stomach; swallow it at noon and in the evening directly or with rice beverage respectively. The eye diseases like fulminant red eye due to wind toxin, blurred vision, dryness of eyes, pain and itch of eyes can be cured with 3 doses in 2 or 3 days. Long term taking of it will cure internal and external visual obstruction. Sexual activity, toxic substance, and food that causes excessive internal heat should be forbidden during the medicine taking period. It is forbidden to use acupuncture and cautery therapy on the head, and to take Zaojiao［皂角, Gleditsia, Gleditsiae Fructus］ and Qianniu［牵牛, Morning Glory, Pharbitis nil（L.）Choisy］ for quick effect when treating eye diseases because they will cause great in jury to the eye.

治老人春时胸膈不利，痰壅气噎，及咽喉诸疾。黍粘汤方。

Shuzhantang Fang（Great Burdock Achene Decoction）is used to treat inhibited chest and diaphragm, to relieve stagnation of phlegm and qi, and various diseases in throat of the aged in spring.

黍粘子三两，炒令香熟　甘草炙，半两

It is composed of 3 Liang of Shuzhanzi［黍粘子, Great Burdock Achene, Fructus Arctii］ that is fried well, and 0.5 Liang of Gancao［甘草, Liquorice Root, Radix Glycyrrhizae］stir-fried.

上为末，捣罗细末。每服一钱，食后、临卧，如常点之。

Pound the above ingredients into powder. Take one Qian of it each time after meal and before sleep. Take it on time.

夏时摄养第十

Chapter 10 Health Preservation in Summer

夏时属火，主于长养。夏心气旺，心主火，味属苦，火能克金。金属肺腑，主辛，其饮食之味，当夏之时，宜减苦增辛，以养肺气。心气盛者，调呵气以疏之。顺之则安，逆之则太阳不长，心气内洞。

Summer pertains to fire, representing the growth and development. Heart qi of people is abundant in summer. Heart corresponds to fire, bitter in taste, and fire restricts metal. Metal belongs to lung, pungent in taste. In summer, therefore, bitterness should be reduced and pungency should be increased in order to nourish lung qi. For people with excessive heart qi, they can use breathing exercise to regulate qi. Following the way ensures life while violating of it will prevent heart qi from developing, resulting in deficiency of it.

盛夏之月，最难治摄。阴气内伏，暑毒外蒸，纵意当风，任性食冷，故人多暴泄之患。

It is the most difficult to preserve health in summer months. As yin qi is latent and steaming summerheat invades from outside, people who like to relax in cool places and indulge themselves in taking cold food are likely to have fulminant diarrhea.

惟是老人尤宜保护：若檐下过道，穿隙破窗，皆不可纳凉。此为贼风，中人暴毒。宜居虚堂净室，水次木阴，洁净之处，自有清凉。

The aged should be cared more seriously. They can not enjoy the cool under the eaves, in the corridor, or by the broken windows because they are easy to be attacked by pathogenic exogenous factors in these places and get sudden and violent stroke. The aged had better live in spacious and clean rooms near to water and shade of trees, which are cool and refreshing naturally.

每日凌晨，进温平顺气汤散一服。饮食温软，不令太饱，畏日长永，但时复进之。渴宜饮粟米温饮、豆蔻熟水。生冷肥腻，尤宜减之。缘老人气弱，当夏之时，纳阴在内，以阴弱之腹，当冷肥之物，则多成滑泄。一伤正气，卒难补复，切宜慎之。若须要食瓜果之类，量虚实少为进之。缘老人思食之物，若有违阻，意便不乐，但随意与之，才食之际，以方便之言解之，往往知味便休，不逆其意，自无所损。

Take a dose of warm and mild Shunqi Tang（Qi Normalizing Decoction）every early morning. The diet of the aged should be warm and soft. Do not let them overeat. Let them eat frequently in proper amount in the long days of summer. It is suitable for the thirsty aged to take warm millet porridge and cardamom decoction instead of raw, cold, fat and greasy food.

It is because that the aged are of qi deficiency in summer and their internal organs store insufficient yin which may lead to diarrhea when taking cold and fat food. In this case the healthy qi is damaged and is difficult to restore in a short time, so great attention should be given to this point. If the aged want to eat fruits like melons, the proper amount should be prepared less than those needed. It is because the aged may be unhappy if they are not provided with the food they want. At this moment, they can be informed about the side effect and the necessity to taste a little instead of overeating. It is a good way to dissuade the aged without going against his will and impairing his health.

若是气弱老人，夏至以后，宜服不燥热、平补肾气暖药三二十服，以助元气，若苁蓉丸、八味丸之类。

For the aged with qi deficiency, after the Summer Solstice, it is advisable to take twenty to thirty doses of neutral formulas to warm and tonify the kidney qi and strengthen the primordial qi, such as Congrong Wan（Cistanche Pill）, Bawei Wan（Eight-Ingredient Pill）and the like.

宜往洁雅寺院中，择虚敞处，以其所好之物悦之。若要寝息，但任其意，不可令久眠。但时时令歇，久则神昏，直召年高相协之人，日陪闲话，论往昔之事，自然喜悦，忘其暑毒。细汤名茶，时为进之，晚凉方归。

It is advisable to accompany the aged to the temple that is clean and elegant, choose a ventilated and spacious place, and please them with what they like. Let them rest if they like but don't let them sleep for a long time.

The frequent rest may make the aged feel dazed so it is advisable to invite some seniors with similar interest to chat and talk about the past. Naturally, they will be happy and forget the summer heat. They should be served with fine soup and famous tea frequently and escorted home in the evening when it is cool.

谨选夏时汤药如后。

The decoctions that can be used in summer are listed below.

夏时用药诸方

Formulas for the Aged in Summer

治老人夏多冷气发动，胸膈气滞，噎塞，脾胃不和，可思饮食。豆蔻散。

Doukou San (Cardamom Powder) is used to treat cold pathogen, stagnation of qi in the chest and diaphragm, choke, incoordination between the spleen and stomach, and anorexia of the aged in summer.

草豆蔻四两，以姜四两炒香黄为度，和姜用　大麦蘖子十两，炒黄　神曲四两，炒黄　杏仁四两，去尖，炒熟　甘草四两，炙　干姜二两，炮制

It is composed to 4 Liang of Caodoukou [草豆蔻, Katsumada Galangal Seed, Semen Alpiniae Katsumadai] fried and mixed with 4 Liang of ginger, 10 Liang of Damainiezi [大麦蘖子, Barley Sprout, Hordei Fructus Germinatus] fried to brown, 4 Liang of Shenqu [神曲, Medicated Leaven,

Massa Medicata Fermentata〕fried to brown, 4 Liang of Xingren〔杏仁, Bitter Apricot Seed, Semen Armeniacae Amarum〕fried well with the pith removed, 4 Liang of Gancao〔甘草, Liquorice Root, Radix Glycyrrhizae〕roasted, and 2 Liang of dried ginger processed.

上为末。每服一钱，如茶点之，不计时候服。

Pound the above ingredients into powder. Take one Qian each time. Take it anytime with some tea.

治老人，夏月宜服，平补下元，明目。苁蓉丸。

Congrong Wan（Cistanche Pill）is used to warm and tonify kidney qi, and improve vision of the aged in summer months.

苁蓉四两　巴戟二两　菊花二两　枸杞子二两

It is composed of 4 Liang of Congrong〔苁蓉, Cistanche, Cistanches Herba〕, 2 Liang of Baji〔巴戟, Morinda Root, Radix Morindae Officinalis〕, 2 Liang of Juhua〔菊花, Chrysanthemums, Dendranthema Morifolium Tzvel.〕, and 2 Liang of Gouqizi〔枸杞子, Lycium, Lycii Fructus〕.

上为末，炼蜜为丸，桐子大。每服，盐汤下二十丸。

Pound the above ingredients into powder. Process it with honey into pills as big as firmiana seeds. Take 20 pills each time with weak brine.

治老人夏月暴发腹痛及泄泻。木香丸。

Muxiang Wan (Costusroot Pill) is used to treat sudden abdominal pain and diarrhea in summer months.

轻好全干蝎二十个，每个擘三两段子，于慢火上炒令黄熟　拣好胡椒三百粒，生　木香一分

Prepare 20 good and complete Ganxie［干蝎, Scorpion, Scorpio］. Split them into 2 or 3 parts. Fry them to brown with slow fire. Select 300 good and fresh Hujiao［胡椒, Pepper, Piperis Fructus］, and prepare 1 Fen of Muxiang［木香, Root of Common Aucklandia, Radix Aucklandiae］.

上件，同药捣为末，湿纸裹烧，粟米饭为丸，如绿豆大。如患腹痛，每服十五丸，煎灯心、称橘皮，生姜汤下。大便不调及泄泻，每服十五丸，煎陈橘皮汤下。

Pound the above ingredients into powder. Wrap them in dampened paper and burn them. Mix them with millet into pills as big as mung beans. For patients with abdominal pain, it is advisable to take 15 pills with fried Dengxin［灯心, Juncus, Junci Medulla］or Jupi［橘皮, Tangerine Peel, Citri Reticulatae Pericarpium］, and fresh ginger decoction. For patients with loose stool and diarrhea, it is advisable to take 15 pills with fried tangerine peel decoction.

治老人夏月，脾胃忽生冷气，心腹胀满疼闷，泄泻不止。诃子散。

Hezi San (Cheubule Powder) is used to treat sudden cold pathogen in the spleen and stomach, fullness, distension and stuffy pain in the heart and abdomen, and persistent diarrhea of the aged in summer months.

诃子皮五个　大腹五个，去皮　甘草半两，炙　白术半两，微炒　草豆蔻十四个，用面裹，烧令面熟黄，去面并皮用　人参去芦头，半两

It is composed of 5 Hezi［诃子, Medicine Terminalia Fruit, Fructus Chebulae］, 5 Dafu［大腹, Areca Peel, Pericarpium Arecae］ with the external skin removed, 0.5 Liang of Gancao［甘草, Liquorice Root, Radix Glycyrrhizae］ stir-fried, 0.5 Liang of Baizhu［白术, Argehead Atractylodes Rhizome, Rhizoma Atractylodis Macrocephalae］ fried slightly, 14 Caodoukou［草豆蔻, Katsumada Galangal Seed, Semen Alpiniae Katsumadai］ wrapped with flour and burnt to brown which is used with the flour and skin removed, and 0.5 Liang of Renshen［人参, Ginseng, Radix Ginseng］ with the top removed.

上为末。每服二钱，水一盏，入生姜少许，枣二个，同煎至六分，去滓，温服。

Pound the above ingredients into powder. Take 2 Qian each time. Put the powder, a little fresh ginger and 2 Chinese dates in a cup of water. Decoct until three fifths is left. Remove the dreg and take the decoction when it is warm.

治老人夏月因食冷，气积滞，或心腹疼痛等，宜常服。

Lengshu San（Scirpus and Zedoray Rhizome Powder）is used to treat stagnation of qi due to intake of cold food in summer, and pains in the heart and abdomen, which is suitable to take regularly.

荆三棱三两，湿纸裹，煨熟透，别杵　蓬莪术二两，同上　乌药二两　益智去皮，二两　甘草三两，炙　陈橘皮二两，用厚朴亦得

The formula is composed of 3 Liang of Jingsanleng［荆三棱, Scirpus, Scirpi Fluviatilis Rhizoma］wrapped in dampened paper and then simmered without pestling, 2 Liang of Peng'eshu［蓬莪术, Curcuma Rhizome, Curcumae Rhizoma］processed in the same way as that of Jingsanleng［荆三棱, Scirpus, Scirpi Fluviatilis Rhizoma］, 2 Liang of Wuyao［乌药, Lindera Root, Linderae Radix］, 2 Liang of Yizhi［益智, Sharp-leaf Glangal Fruit, Fructus Alpiniae Oxyphyllae］with the skin removed, 3 Liang of Gancao［甘草, Liquorice Root, Radix Glycyrrhizae］stir-fried, and 2 Liang of Chenjupi［陈橘皮, Dried Tangerine Peel, Pericarpium Citri Reticulatae］or Houpu［厚朴, Magnolia Bark, Cortex Magnoliae Officinalis］.

上为末。每服入盐点之，不计时候，一钱。

Pound the above ingredients into powder. Take one Qian each time. Take it anytime with some brine.

治老人，夏月宜服三圣丸，祛逐风冷气，进食和胃，去痰滞，腰膝冷痛。

Sansheng Wan（Pill of Three Effective Medicinals）is used to expel wind pathogen and cold qi, improve appetite, harmonize the stomach, remove phlegm stagnation and cold pain in the lumbus and knees of the aged in summer.

威灵仙净洗，去土，拣择，焙干，秤五两　干姜二两，炮制　乌头二两，炮制，去皮脐，秤

It is composed of 5 Liang of Weilingxian ［威灵仙, Clematis, Clematidis Radix］ washed, dried, and weighed with the earth removed, 2 Liang of dried ginger processed, and 2 Liang of Wutou ［乌头, Common Monkshood, Aconitum carmichaeli Debx.］ processed and weighed with the skin and navel removed.

上件为末，煮枣肉为丸，如梧子大。每服十五丸至二十丸，温姜汤下。

Pound the above ingredients into powder. Process it with Chinese dates into pills as big as firmiana seeds. Take 15 to 20 pills each time with warm ginger decoction.

治老人，夏月宜服平补楮实丸方。驻颜壮筋骨，补益元藏，疗积冷虚乏，一切气疾。暖胃，进酒食，久服令人轻健，此神效方。

Chushi Wan（Permulberry Fruit Pill）is used to nourish the aged in summer months, to keep agerasia, strengthen the sinews and bones, tonify kidney qi, treat deficiency and lassitude due to the accumulated cold, and all qi diseases. It is effective to warm the stomach and improve appetite. Long-term taking of it will relax and refresh the body.

楮实半斤，轻杵，去白及膜，拣择净，微微炒　鹿茸四两，茄子茸为上，其次亦

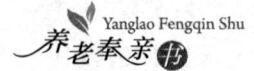

得净瓮上炙令黄色，如无，则鹿角屑代之亦妙　大附子四两，炮，去皮脐，出火毒　怀州牛膝四两，去芦头，酒浸二宿，焙　紫巴戟四两，洗，去心　金钗石斛四两，去根，拣净，细细切之　川干姜二两，炮制，急于新水内净过　肉桂二两，去粗皮

　　It is composed of 0.5 Jin of Chushi［楮实，Papermulberry Fruit, Fructus Broussonetiae］pestled and fried slightly with the clean ones selected after the white part and membrane being removed, 4 Liang of Lurong［鹿茸，Pilose Antler, Cornu Cervi Pantotrichum］or the young pilose antler or Lujiaoxie［鹿角屑，Deer Antler Flakes, Cervi Cornu in Frustis］stir-fried to brown on a clean jar, 4 Liang of big Fuzi［附子，Aconite, Radix Aconiti Praeparata］processed with the skin and navel and heat toxin removed, 4 Liang of Niuxi［牛膝，Twotoothed Achyranthes Root, Radix Achyranthis Bidentatae］from Huaizhou with the top removed, steeped in liquor for 2 nights and baked, 4 Liang of purple Baji［巴戟，Morinda Root, Radix Morindae Officinalis］washed with the pith discarded, 4 Liang of Jinchaishihu［金钗石斛，Golden Hairpin Dendrobium, Dendrobii Nobilis Herba］washed and cut thinly after the root of it being removed, 2 Liang of Sichuan dried ginger processed by being washed in clean water, and 2 Liang of Rougui［肉桂，Cassia Bark, Cortex Cinnamomi］with its rough skin removed.

　　上件，八味为末。楮实子一味，用砂盆别研二日，令烂细后，旋入前药末同研拌令细匀，入煮枣内同研拌得所，方入铁臼杵二千下，丸如桐子大。每服三十丸，温酒下。忌牛肉、豉汁。

　　Pound the above 8 ingredients into powder. Grind Chushizi［楮实子，Papermulberry Fruit, Fructus Broussonetiae］in an earthen pot for 2 days separately. After it is in fine powder, add the previous powder and mix them together, then add the boiled Chinese dates and pestle them in iron mortar for 2000 times, making it into pills as big as firmiana seeds. Take 30 pills each time with warm liquor. It is incompatible with beef and fermented soybean juice.

治老人百疾，常服四顺汤。

Sishun Tang（Four Regulation Decoction）is used to treat all kinds of diseases of the aged.

神曲四两，入生姜四两去皮，一处作饼子，焙干　甘草一两半，炙黄　大麦蘗子二两，炒香熟　草豆蔻一两半，先炮熟，去皮细锉用

It is composed of 4 Liang of Shenqu［神曲, Medicated Leaven, Massa Medicata Fermentata］mixed with 4 Liang of fresh ginger with the skin removed and made into pancakes before being baked, 1.5 Liang of Gancao［甘草, Liquorice Root, Radix Glycyrrhizae］stir-fried to brown, 2 Liang of Damainiezi［大麦蘗子, Barley Sprout, Hordei Fructus Germinatus］stir-fried well, and 1.5 Liang of Caodoukou［草豆蔻, Katsumada Galangal Seed, Semen Alpiniae Katsumadai］with the skin removed and then filed after being cooked.

上件为末，盐点之一钱。

Pound the above ingredients into powder with 1 Qian of salt.

妇人年老，夏月平补血海，活血去风。五倍丸。

Wubei Wan（Chinese Gall Pill）is used to nourish thoroughfare vessel, activate blood and expel wind of the aged females in summer months.

五倍子二两　　川芎二两，锉细　　菊花二两　　荆芥穗二两　　旋覆花二两

It is composed of 2 Liang of Wubeizi ［五倍子，Chinese Gall, Galla Chinensis］, 2 Liang of Chuanxiong ［川芎，Sichuan Lovage Rhizome, Ligusticum chuanxiong Hort.］ filed, 2 Liang of Juhua ［菊花，Chrysanthemums, Dendranthema Morifolium Tzvel.］, 2 Liang of Jingjiesui ［荆芥穗，Schizonepeta Spike, Schizonepetae Flos］, and 2 Liang of Xuanfuhua ［旋覆花，Inula Flower, Flos Inula Japonica］.

上为末，蜜为丸如桐子大，每日空心五更，晚食后，盐汤、酒下十五丸。吃至半月日，觉见渐安，手足有力，眼目鲜明，进得饮食，大旺血海。请每一日三服，若见大段安乐，一日只吃一服尤佳。

Pound the above ingredients into powder. Process it with honey into pills as big as firmiana seeds. Take 15 pills with brine and liquor after dinner and before dawn on an empty stomach. After taking it for half a month, the spirit will be tranquillized, the hands and feet will be stronger, the vision will be better, the appetite will be improved, and the thoroughfare vessel will be replenished. Take it 3 times a day. If the patient feels much better for a long period, it is advisable to take only one dose a day.

治老人脾胃弱，不思饮食，吐泻霍乱。理中丸。

Lizhong Wan（Middle-Regulating Pill）is used to treat deficiency in the spleen and stomach, anorexia, vomiting, diarrhea and cholera of the aged.

人参　甘草　干姜　白术各等分

It is composed of Renshen［人参, Ginseng, Radix Ginseng］, Gancao［甘草, Liquorice Root, Radix Glycyrrhizae］, dried ginger and Baizhu［白术, Argehead Atractylodes Rhizome, Rhizoma Atractylodis Macrocephalae］in equal amount respectively.

上为末，炼蜜为丸，桐子大。每服十五丸，食前服。

Pound the above ingredients into powder. Process it with honey into pills as big as firmiana seeds. Take 15 pills each time on an empty stomach.

夏月消食和气。橘红散。

Juhong San（Red Tangerine Peel Powder）is used to promote digestion and harmonize qi in summer months..

陈橘皮一斤半，汤浸洗五七度，用净巾拭干后，用生姜五两，取自然汁，拌橘皮令匀，淹一宿，焙干，秤一斤　肉豆蔻半两　甘草五两

Prepare 1.5 Jin of Chenjupi［陈橘皮, Dried Tangerine Peel, Pericarpium Citri Reticulatae］steeped in hot water for 5 or 7 times and dried with a clean towel. Mix it with fresh ginger juice out of 5 Liang of fresh ginger, steep it for a night, dry it until 1 Jin is left. Prepare 0.5 Liang of Roudoukou［肉豆蔻, Nutmeg, Semen Myristicae］, and 5 Liang of Gancao［甘草,

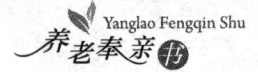

Liquorice Root, Radix Glycyrrhizae〕.

上,先将甘草寸截,用白盐五两一处同炒,候盐红色,甘草赤色为度。一处为末,如茶点之。

Cut the Gancao〔甘草, Liquorice Root, Radix Glycyrrhizae〕into segments. Fry it with 5 Liang of salt till both turning red. Pound the above ingredients into powder. Take it with some tea.

夏月,平胃,补老人元脏虚弱,腑气不顺,壮筋骨,益颜容,固精髓。八仙丸。

Baxian Wan (Pill of Eight Effective Medicinals) is used to calm stomach, replenish the kidney qi, regulate qi stagnation in the fu-organs, strengthen sinews and bones, improve looks, and strengthen essence and marrow of the aged in summer months.

泽泻三两　茯苓二两,去粗皮　牡丹三两　干薯药四两,微炒炙　官桂二两　山茱萸四两　生干地黄八两,洗,干杵　附子三两,炮,去皮脐,研

It is composed of 3 Liang of Zexie〔泽泻, Oriental Waterplantain Rhizome, Rhizoma Alismatis〕, 2 Liang of Fuling〔茯苓, Indian Bread, Poria〕with the rough skin removed, 3 Liang of Mudan〔牡丹, Peony, Cortex Moutan Radicis〕, 4 Liang of dried Shuyao〔薯药, Dioscorea, Dioscoreae Rhizoma〕, 2 Liang of Guangui〔官桂, Cassia Cortex Cinnamomi〕, 4 Liang of Shanzhuyu〔山茱萸, Cornus, Fructus Corni〕, 8 Liang of fresh Gandihuang〔干地黄, Dried Rehmannia, Radix Rehmanniae〕washed, dried and pestled, and

3 Liang of Fuzi［附子, Aconite, Radix Aconiti Praeparata］processed with the skin and navel removed and then ground.

上，事持了焙干，惟桂不焙，为末。炼蜜为丸，如桐子大。每日空心，温酒或盐汤下三十丸。

Dry the above ingredients and bake them excepting Guangui［官桂, Cassia Cortex Cinnamomi］. Pound the above ingredients into powder. Process the powder with honey into pills as big as firmiana seeds. Take 30 pills with warm liquor or brine on an empty stomach each day.

秋时摄养第十一

Chapter 11　Health Preservation in Autumn

秋属金，主于肃杀。秋，肺气旺，肺属金，味属辛，金能克木。木属肝，肝主酸，当秋之时，其饮食之味，宜减辛增酸，以养肝气。肺气盛者，调呬气以泄之。顺之则安，逆之则太阴不收，肺气焦满。

Autumn is the season of the element metal, and it governs purification and suppress. In autumn, the lung qi which is associated with metal thrives, corresponds to pungent flavor, and metal can restrain wood. The wood belongs to liver, and the taste that corresponds to liver is sour. Thus, in autumn one should reduce the taking of pungent food and enhance the sourness in flavor to nourish liver qi. Those with exuberant lung qi should regulate the breath to expel it. Follow the rule and then one will prosper while disobedience of the rule may lead to dysfunction of taiyin meridian and fullness and distention of lung qi.

秋时凄风惨雨，草木黄落。高年之人，身虽老弱，心亦如壮，秋时思念往昔亲朋，动多伤感。季秋之后，水冷草枯，多发宿患，此时人子最宜承奉，晨昏体悉，举止看详。若颜色不乐，便须多方诱说，使役其心神，则忘其秋思。其新登五谷，不宜与食，易动人宿疾。若素知宿患，秋终多发，或痰涎喘嗽，或风眩痹癖，或秘泄劳倦，若寒热进退。计其所发之疾，预于未发已前，择其中和应病之药，预与服食，止其欲发。今布秋时汤药如后。

  Autumn is characterized by bleak weather and the scene of falling leaves and withering grass. While physically weak, the aged is still like the young in mind and likely to miss old friends and relatives, inducing their sorrow and grief. After the last month of the autumn, the water runs cold and the grass withers, in which abiding ailments may reoccur. Thus, people should fulfill their filial obligations and pay close attention to their parents' health from day to night. If the aged is not in good mood, the offspring should soothe them in various ways to help them lift spirit and forget sorrows. The newly-harvested 5 cereals should not be served for the aged to avoid the onset of abiding ailments. The abiding ailments likely to reoccur in autumn include asthmatic cough with phlegm, dizziness, flaccidity, lump in the hypochondrium, constipation, diarrhea, tiredness, severe or slight fever due to aversion to cold. The offspring should be alert to these diseases, take corresponding measures beforehand and prepare appropriate medicinals for the aged to prevent the onset of the diseases. The formulas for the aged used in autumn are listed below.

秋时用药诸方

Formulas for the Aged in Autumn

治老人一切泻利。七宝丹。此药如久患泻痢,诸药疗不差者,服此药无不差。若老人反脾泄滑,大宜服此药。

Qibao Dan (Seven Treasure Pill) can treat all kinds of diarrhea of the aged, especially the chronic diarrhea that is hard to cure for a long time. It is effective to treat severe diarrhea due to disorder of the spleen.

附子炮　当归　陈橘皮　干姜以上各一两　吴茱萸　厚朴以姜汁炙　南椒以上三味各半两　舶上硫黄一两

Take 1 Liang of processed Fuzi [附子, Aconite, Radix Aconiti Praeparatae], 1 Liang of Danggui [当归, Angelica, Radix Angelicae Sinensis], 1 Liang of Chenjupi [陈橘皮, Dried Tangerine Peel, Pericarpium Citri Reticulatae], 1 Liang of dried ginger, half a Liang of Wuzhuyu [吴茱萸, Evodia Fruit, Fructus Evodiae], half a Liang of Houpo [厚朴, Magnolia, Cortex Magnoliae Officinalis] stir-baked with ginger juice, half a Liang of Nanjiao [南椒, Zanthoxylum], half a Liang of sulfur from sea-going vessel.

上件七味,细锉,以慢火焙过,捣罗为末,与硫黄末同拌匀,一处煎,米醋和,作两剂。却以白面半斤,和令得所,亦令分作两剂。用裹药如烧饼法,用文武火煨,令面熟为度。去却面,于臼中捣三百下,丸如桐子大。如患诸般泻痢,以米汤下二十丸,空心日午服。如患气痛及宿冷不消,以姜盐汤下二十丸,空心日午服。如患气痛及宿冷,并无忌。此方如神如圣，其效无及。

Pestle and bake the above ingredients with slow fire, pound them into powder and mix with sulfur powder. Decoct the mixture together with rice vinegar into 2 portions. Take half a Jin of wheat flour and make into 2 pastes. Wrap the mixture with the paste like making Chinese pancake, bake it with strong and gentle fire alternately until it is cooked. After that, remove the paste and pound it about 300 times in a mortar to make it into pills as big as firmiana seeds. To treat various diarrhea, take 20 pills with rice soup at noon before meal. To treat pain due to qi disorder and lingering cold from sleep, take 20 pills with ginger and salt soup at noon on an empty stomach, which is not contraindicated with anything. This formula is very effective for the aged.

治老人乘秋，脏腑虚冷，滑泄不定。摄脾丸。

Shepi Wan（Spleen-Fortifying Pill）can deal with deficiency-cold in zang-fu organs and diarrhea of the aged.

木香　诃子炮，去核　厚朴生姜汁炙　五倍子　白术各等分

It is composed of Muxiang［木香, Costusroot, Radix Aucklandiae］, Hezi［诃子, Terminalia, Fructus Chebulae］processed and with the core removed, Houpo［厚朴, Magnolia, Cortex Magnoliae Officinalis］fried with fresh ginger juice, Wubeizi［五倍子, Gallnut, Galla Chinensis］, and Baizhu［白术, Atractylodes, Rhizoma Atractylodis Macrocephalae］in equal amount respectively.

上为末，用烧粟米饭为丸桐子大。每服十丸，米饮送下。

Pound the above ingredients into powder, mix with the millet rice and make them into pills as large as firmiana seeds. Take 10 pills each time with rice beverage.

治老人秋肺壅滞，涎嗽闲作，胃脘痰滞，塞闷不快。威灵仙丸。

Weilingxian Wan（Clematis Root Pill）can be used to treat lung obstruction in autumn, cough due to saliva disorder, phlegm retention in the stomach, depression due to lump in the abdomen for the aged.

威灵仙洗择去土，焙干为末，四两　干薄荷取末，一两　皂角一斤，不蛀肥者，以河水浸洗，去黑皮，用银石器内，用河水软揉，去滓，绢滤去粗，熬成膏

Take 4 Liang of Weilingxian［威灵仙, Clematis Root, Radix Clematidis］that is washed, removed of mud and baked into powder, 1 Liang of dry Bohe［薄荷, Mint, Herba Menthae］ground into powder, and 1 Liang of Zaojiao［皂角, Chinese honeylocust fruit, Spina Gleditsiae］that is not damaged by worms. Wash Zaojiao in the river to remove the black skin and knead it soft with the river water in the silver mortar, remove the dregs and filter the impurities with silk, boil it into paste.

上入前膏，搜丸如桐子大。每服三十丸，临卧生姜汤吞下。

Decoct the above 3 ingredients into paste and make them into pills as big as firmiana seeds. Take 30 pills each time with fresh ginger soup before going to bed.

治老人脾脏泄泻，中心气不和，精神倦怠，不思饮食。神授高青丸。

Gaoqing Wan（Galangal and Aristolochia Pill）can treat diarrhea due to spleen deficiency, harmonize the stomach and spleen, treat lassitude and poor appetite for the aged.

高良姜　青木香各一两

Take 1 Liang of Gaoliangjiang［高良姜, Lesser Galangal Rhizome, Rhizoma Alpiniae Officinarum］and 1 Liang of Qingmuxiang［青木香, Aristolochia Root, Radix Aristolochiae］.

上二味为末，煮枣肉为丸，桐子大。干姜汤下十五丸至二十丸。

Pound the above 2 ingredients into powder, mix it with Chinese dates and boil into pills as big as firmiana seeds. Take 15–20 pills with dried ginger soup.

治老人秋后多发嗽，远年一切嗽疾，并劳嗽痰壅。保救丹。

Baojiu Dan（Cough Suppressing Pill）can deal with the recurrent cough, abiding cough and pulmonary cough due to phlegm stagnation for the aged.

蛤蚧一个，如是丈夫患，取腰前一截雄者用之；女人患，取雌者腰后一截用之　不蛀皂角二挺，涂酥炙，去黑皮并子　干地黄一分，熟蒸如饧　五味子一分　杏仁一分，去皮尖，用童子小便浸一伏时，入蜜，炒黄色　半夏一分，浆水煮三七遍　丁香少许

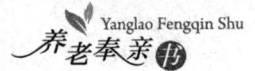

Prepare a gecko, select the front part of a male gecko's waist for a male patient, the rear part of a female gecko's waist for a femaile patient. Prepare 2 Zaojiao［皂角，Chinese honeylocust fruit, Spina Gleditsiae］undamaged by worms, fry it with butter and remove the black skin and seed. Prepare 1 Fen of Gandihuang［干地黄，Dried Rehmannia, Radix Rehmanniae］steamed and cooked as soft as malt syrup. Prepare 1 Fen of Wuweizi［五味子，Shizandra, Fructus Schisandrae］. Prepare 1 Fen of Xingren［杏仁，Apricot Seed, Semen Armeniaccae Amarum］with its tip and skin removed, soak it in boy urine for a day and stir-fry it with honey until it is yellow in color. Prepare 1 Fen of Banxia［半夏，Ternate, Rhizoma Pinelliae］boiled in millet soup for 3 to 7 times and a bit of Dingxiang［丁香，Clove, Flos Syzygii Aromatici］.

上为末，炼蜜为丸，如桐子大。每日食前一服，五丸姜汤下。

Pound the above ingredients into powder, mix with honey and make them into pills as big as firmiana seeds. Take 5 pills with ginger soup each day before meal.

治老人膈滞，肺疾痰嗽。生姜汤。

Shengjiang Tang（Fresh Ginger Decoction）can treat the diaphragm stagnation and cough with phlegm due to lung diseases for the aged.

杏仁四两，去皮尖　生姜六两，去皮，细横切之　甘草三分　桃仁半两，去皮尖　盐花三两

Prepare 4 Liang of Xingren［杏仁，Apricot Seed，Semen Armeniaccae

Amarum〕with its tip and skin removed, 6 Liang of Shengjiang〔生姜, Raw Ginger, Rhizoma Zingiberis Recens〕with its skin peeled and sliced into shreds, 3 Fen of Gancao〔甘草, liquorice, Radix Glycyrrhizae〕, 0.5 Liang of Taoren〔桃仁, Peach Seed, Semen Perisicae〕with the tip and skin removed, 3 Liang of salt.

上，以杏仁、桃仁、姜、湿纸同裹煨，沙盆内研极细后，入甘草、盐再研，洁器贮之，汤点服。

Wrap the above mentioned Xingren〔杏仁, Apricot Seed, Semen Armeniaccae Amarum〕, Taoren〔桃仁, Peach Seed, Semen Perisicae〕and ginger in wet tissue, simmer it and then pound it finely in a basin. Add Gancao〔甘草, Liquorice, Radix Glycyrrhizae〕and salt and pound again. Store it in a clean container and take a small amount each time with hot water.

治诸般腹泻不止，及年高久泻。健脾散。

Jianpi San (Spleen Invigorating Powder) can treat various severe and chronic diarrhea of the aged.

川乌头炮，去皮脐，三分　厚朴去皮，姜汁制　甘草炙　干姜炮，各一两

Prepare 3 Fen of Chuanwutou〔川乌头, Aconite Main Root, Aconitumcarmichaeli Debx〕processed and with its skin and umbilicus removed, one Liang of Houpo〔厚朴, Magnolia, Cortex Magnoliae Officinalis〕with its skin peeled and processed with ginger juice, 1 Liang of dried ginger processed, and 1 Liang of Gancao〔甘草, Liquorice, Radix Glycyrrhizae〕stir-fried.

上为末。每服一钱，水三合，生姜二片，煎至二合，热服。并进二服，立止。

Pound the above ingredients into powder. Take 1 Qian each time, mix it with 3 He of water and 2 pieces of fresh ginger, decoct until 2 He is left. Take 2 dosages at one time when it is hot and the diarrhea can be relieved immediately.

冬时摄养第十二

Chapter 12　Health Preservation in Winter

冬属水，主于敛藏。冬肾气旺，属水，味属咸。水克火，火属心，心主苦。当冬之时，其饮食之味，宜减咸而增苦，以养心气。肾气盛者，调吹气以平之。顺之则安，逆之则少阴不藏，肾之水独沉。

Winter is the season of the element water and governs storage. In winter, the kidney qi is in dominance, which belongs to water element and corresponds to salty flavor. Water restrains fire and fire belongs to heart, and heart corresponds to bitterness. When winter comes, one should reduce the salty flavor and increase the bitterness in diet to nourish heart qi. For those with exuberant kidney qi, they should regulate the breath to balance it. Those who follow the rules will be healthy while disobedience will lead to lesser yin syndrome and descending of kidney qi.

三冬之月，最宜居处密室，温暖衾服，调其饮食，适其寒温。大寒之日，山药酒、肉酒时进一杯，以扶衰弱，以御寒气，不可轻出，触冒寒风。缘老人血气虚怯，真阳气少，若感寒邪，便成疾患，多为嗽、吐逆、

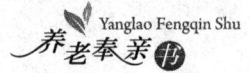

麻痹、昏眩之疾。冬燥，煎炉之物尤宜少食。冬月阳气在内，阴气在外，池沼之中，冰坚如石，地裂横璺，寒从下起，人亦如是。故盛冬月，人多患膈气满急之疾，老人多有上热下冷之患。如冬月阳气在内，虚阳上攻，若食炙煿燥热之物，故多有壅、噎、痰嗽、眼目之疾。亦不宜澡沐，阳气内蕴之时，若加汤火所逼，须出大汗。高年阳气发泄，骨肉疏薄，易于伤动，多感外疾。惟早眠晚起，以避霜威。晨朝宜饮少醇酒，然后进粥。临卧，宜服微凉膈化痰药一服。

In winter, it is recommended to stay at home wearing warm clothes and regulate the diet to deal with coldness. On the day of the Great Cold, the elderly people should take tonic diet made of yam, meat and wine from time to time to strengthen body resistance and defend against cold qi. They should not go outside if not necessary to avoid the risk of wind and cold damage. It is because that the elderly are deficient in blood and qi especially genuine yang qi. If caught with cold-pathogen, they would suffer from diseases like cough, vomiting, paralysis and dizziness. It is suggested to take less grilled and fried food in winter because of the dry weather. In winter, yang qi is stored internally while yin qi is exposed externally, which is characterized by hard-frozen ice in the pond, swamp and frost-cracked earth. The coldness in winter travels from the bottom to the top and so does human beings. Thus, in the coldest month of winter, people are likely to suffer from asthmatic diseases due to fullness of diaphragm, and the aged tend to suffer from coldness in the lower body and heat in the upper one. In winter, yang qi stays inside and sufficient yang may go upward, so diseases like stasis, choke, cough with phlegm and eye disorder may occur if people take roasted, dry and hot food. And it is also not recommended for the elderly to bath in winter because the induced sweating may discharge and damage their yang qi and lead to fracture and cold damage due to invasion of exogenous pathogens. They should sleep early and get up late to avoid cold related damage; drink a little mellow wine and take some porridge in the morning and take a dose of medicines that can cool the diaphragm and dissipate phlegm before going to bed.

今列冬时汤药如后。

The formulas for the aged to take in winter are listed below.

冬时用药诸方
Formulas for the Aged in Winter

治老人大肠风燥气秘。陈橘丸（霍大使与冯尚药同定此方）。

Chenju Wan (Tangerine Peel Pill) can treat constipation due to wind-dryness in large intestine for the aged. (Huo Dashi and Feng Shangyao co-created this formula)

陈橘皮去瓤，一两　槟榔细锉，半两　木香一分　羌活去芦头，半两　防风去芦头，半两　青皮子去瓤，半两　枳壳面炒，去瓤，半两　不蛀皂角两挺，去黑皮，酥炙黄　郁李仁一两，去皮尖，炒黄　牵牛微炒，杵细，罗，取末，二两

Prepare one Liang of Chenjupi [陈橘皮, Dried Tangerine Peel, Pericarpium Citri Reticulatae] with its pulp removed, half a Liang of Binglang [槟榔, Areca Seed, Semen Arecae] sliced into thin pieces, one Fen of Muxiang

［木香，Costusroot, Radix Aucklandiae］half a Liang of Qianghuo ［羌活，Angelica polyclada, Rhizoma seu Radix Notopterygii］with its rhizome and top removed, half a Liang of Fangfeng ［防风，Anisomeles, Radix Ledebouriellae］with its rhizome and top removed, half a Liang of Qingpizi ［青皮子，Green Tangerine Peel, Pericarpium Citri Reticulatae Viride］with its pulp removed, half a Liang of Zhike ［枳壳，Bitter Orange, Fructus Aurantii］with its pulp removed and stir-fried with flour, 2 pieces of Zaojiao ［皂角，Chinese Honeylocust Fruit, Spina Gleditsiae］undamaged by worms and with their black skin peeled and fried to brown, one Liang of Yuliren ［郁李仁，Chinese Dwarf Cherry, Seed Semen Pruni］with its skin and top removed and stir-fried to brown, 2 Liang of Qianniu ［牵牛，Morning Glory, Pharbitidis］stir-fried slightly, pounded, filtered to get the powder.

上为末，郁李仁、牵牛同研拌匀，炼蜜为丸，桐子大。每服二十丸，食前用姜汤下。未利，渐加三十丸，以利为度。

Pound the above ingredients and mix with the powder of the Yuliren［郁李仁，Chinese Dwarf Cherry, Seed Semen Pruni］and Qianniu ［牵牛，Morning Glory, Pharbitidis］, make it into pills as big as firmiana seeds with processed honey. Take 20 pills each time with ginger soup before meal. If the effect is not desirable, increase the dosage to 30 pills each time until the constipation is relieved.

老人有热，壅滞不快，大肠时秘结，诸热毒生疮。搜风顺气。牵牛丸。

Qianniu Wan（Morning Glory Pill）is used to treat stasis, constipation and sore ulcer due to heat toxin for the aged by tracking the wind pathogen and guiding qi downward.

牵牛二两，饭甑蒸过　木通一两　青橘一两，去穰　桑白皮一两　赤芍药一两　木香半两

Prepare 2 Liang of steamed Qianniu ［牵牛，Morningglory, Pharbitidis］, one Liang of Mutong ［木通，Akebia Stem, Caulis Akebiae］, one Liang of Qingju ［青橘，Green Mandarin, Citrus Nobilis］ with its pulp removed, one Liang of Sangbaipi ［桑白皮，Mulferry Root Bark, Cortex Mori Radicis］, one Liang of Chishaoyao ［赤芍药，Red Peony, Radix Paeoniae Rubra］, half a Liang of Muxiang ［木香，Costusroot, Radix Aucklandiae］.

上为末，炼蜜为丸，如桐子大。每服十五丸至二十丸，丈夫酒下；妇人血气，醋汤下。

Pound the above ingredients into powder and make them into pills as big as firmiana seeds with processed honey. Male patients can take 15-20 pills with wine while the female patients can take them with vinegar soup to treat blood diseases.

解老人热秘方。大附子一个，烧留性，研为末。每服一钱，热酒调下。

Here is a secret formula for treating heat syndrome of the aged. Prepare one big Fuzi ［附子，Aconite, Radix Aconiti Praeparatae］, scorch it but do not impair its property, pestle it into powder and take 1 Qian each time with hot wine.

食治养老序第十三

Chapter 13 Preface to the Support of the Aged with Diet Therapy

昔圣人诠置药石，疗诸疾病者，以其五脏本于五行，五行有相生胜之理。荣卫本于阴阳，阴阳有逆顺之理也。故万物皆禀阴阳五行而生，有五色焉，有五味焉，有寒热焉，有良毒焉。人取其色味冷热良毒之性，归之五行，处以为药，以治诸疾。顺五行之气者，以相生之物为药以养之；逆五行之气者，以相胜之物为药以攻之。或泻母以利子，或益子以补母，此用药之奇法也。

Medical sages in ancient times explained the reason for applying medicinal herbs and stone needles in treating various diseases being that the 5 zang-organs correspond to the 5 elements and the 5 elements generate and restrict each other on one aspect, the nutrient qi and the defensive qi pertain to yin and yang, and yin and yang oppose and depend on each other on the other aspect. Therefore, all things in nature are endowed with life in accordance with yin and yang and the 5 elements, whose properties are classified based on the 5 colors, the 5 kinds of seasonings, cold and heat, toxic and nontoxic. Medical sages attributed these properties to the five elements and applied them in medication to treat various diseases. For those that correspond with the regular order of the five elements, their generating element can be taken as medicinals to nourish them; for those that go against with the regular order of the five elements, their restricting element can be taken as medicinals to treat them. There are still some other effective methods like benefiting the child-organ by purging the mother-organ and tonifying the mother-organ by reinforcing the child-organ.

《经》曰：天地，万物之盗。人，万物之盗。人，所以盗万物为资养之法。其水陆之物为饮食者不啻千品，其五色、五味、冷热、补泻之性，亦皆禀于阴阳五行，与药无殊。大体用药之法，以冷治热，以热治冷，实则泻之，虚则补之，此用药之大要也。人若能知其食性，调而用之，则倍胜于药也。

Jing（*Huangdi's Canon of Implicit Conjunction*）says: All the things in nature take advantage of the yin and yang to come into being, and human beings are nurtured by all the things in nature to exist. Human beings make use of all the things in nature to cultivate and nourish themselves. The variety of foods from land and water is more than 1000, and their properties, like pertaining to the 5 colors, the 5 kinds of seasonings, cold and heat, possessing tonifying and purging action, are all based on the yin and yang and the five elements, very similar with those of medicinals. The guiding principle for using medicinals is to treat heat syndrome with herbs cold in nature, treat cold syndrome with herbs heat in nature, treat excess syndrome with purging method, treat deficiency syndrome with tonifying method. If the properties of foods can be identified and adopted to treat diseases, their curative effect would be much better than the medicinals.

缘老人之性，皆厌于药而喜于食，以食治疾，胜于用药。况是老人之疾，慎于吐利，尤宜食以治之。凡老人有患，宜先以食治，食治未愈，然后命药，此养老人之大法也。是以善治病者，不如善慎疾；善治药者，不如善治食。今以《食医心镜》《食疗本草》《诠食要法》《诸家法馔》及《太平圣惠方》食治诸法，类成养老食治方。各开门目，用治诸疾，具列于下。为人子者，宜留意焉。

承奉郎前守泰州兴化县令　陈直述

The aged are mostly in favor of foods rather than medicinals to treat diseases. So it is better to treat diseases with foods instead of medicinals for the aged. Besides, it should be cautious to avoid vomiting and dysentery when treating diseases of the aged and diet therapy is especially appropriate for them. To treat the aged, diet therapy is preferred firstly and if uncured, medicinals can be used then. This is an important principle for cultivating the health of the aged. Therefore, the physicians who are good at preventing diseases are better than those who are good at treating diseases; those who are good at treating diseases with diet therapy are better than those who are good at treating diseases with medicinals. This book collected and classified dietotherapy formulas from *Shiyi Xinjing*（*Heart Mirror of Dietotherapy*）, *Shiliao Bencao*（*Materia Medica for Dietotherapy*）, *Quanshi Yaofa*（*Essential Methods for Food Therapy*）, *Zhujia Fazhuan*（*Food Preparation Methods of Various Schools*）, *Taiping*

Shenghui Fang (*Taiping Holy Prescriptions for Universal Relief*), and compiled them together to support the aged. The formulas are grouped into respective categories and the diseases they are expected to treat are listed accordingly. Those who have elderly parents are supposed to show more concern over them.

Chen Zhi,

Chengfeng Lang (an ancient official title), Magistrate of Xinghua county, Taizhou city

食治老人诸疾方第十四

Chapter 14　Formulas to Treat Various Diseases of the Aged with Diet Therapy

食治养老益气方
Formulas to Support the Aged and Benefit Qi with Diet Therapy

食治老人补虚。益气牛乳方。

Yiqi Niuru Fang（Milk Formula to Benefit Qi）is used to tonify deficiency of the aged.

牛乳五升　荜茇末一两

Prepare 5 Sheng of milk and 1 Liang of Biji ［荜茇, Long Pepper, Piper Longum L.］.

上件药入银器内，以水三升，和乳合煎，取三升后入瓷合中，每于食前暖一小盏服之。

Put the above ingredients into silverware. Mix 3 Sheng of water with the milk. Boil until 3 Sheng is left and put it into the porcelain ware. Warm one small cup of it and take it before meals.

食治老人补虚羸乏气力。法制猪肚方。
Fazhi Zhudu Fang（Boiled Pork Tripe Formula）can be used to treat weakness, emaciation, and deficiency of qi and strength.

獖猪肚一枚洗，如食法　人参半两，去芦头　干姜二钱，炮制，锉　椒二钱，去目，不开口者，微炒，去汗　葱白七茎，去须，切　糯米二合

Take 1 tripe of neutered pig and wash clean like the way before serving. Take 0.5 Liang of Renshen ［人参, Ginseng, Ginseng Radix］ and remove the top. Take 2 Qian of dried ginger, process and grind it into powder with a file. Take 2 Qian of Jiao ［椒, Zanthoxylum, Zanthoxyli Pericarpium］, have the seeds and unsplit ones taken out, then stir-fry slightly. Take 7 pieces of scallion, remove the root and slice them. Prepare 2 He of glutinous rice.

上件捣为末。入米合和相得，入猪肚内，缝合，勿令泄气。以水五升于铛内，微火煮令烂熟。空心服，放温服之。次，暖酒一中盏饮之。
Grind the above ingredients into powder and mix them with the sticky rice. Put them into the pork tripe, sew up and make it airtight. Fill the wok with 5 Sheng of water, simmer it until it is well cooked. Take it warm on an empty stomach. Take it with a medium cup of lukewarm wine on the second dose.

老人益气牛乳方。牛乳最宜老人，平补血脉，益心，长肌肉，令人

身体康强润泽，面目光悦，志不衰。故为人子者，常须供之，以为常食。或为乳饼，或作断乳等，恒使恣意充足为度，此物胜肉远矣。

Laoren Yiqi Niuru Fang（Qi-Benefiting Milk Formula for the Aged）. Milk is the optimum food for the aged. It is neutral in nature and it nourishes the blood and vessels, benefits the heart, engenders muscles, keeps the body strong, skin moist, complexion lustrous and mind agile. People need to supply their parents with milk regularly. Milk can be made into cookies or replace human milk, and it ought to be kept available all the time since it is more nutritious than meat.

食治老人养老，以药水饮牛，取乳服食方。

Quru Fushi Fang（Formula of Taking Milk Produced by Cow Fed with Medicinals）is to feed cows with medicinals and take the milk produced by them.

钟乳一斤，上好者细研　人参三两，去芦头　甘草五两，炙微赤，锉　干地黄三两　黄芪二两，锉　杜仲三两，去皱皮用　肉苁蓉六两　白茯苓五两　麦门冬四两，去心　薯蓣六两　石斛二两，去根锉

Prepare 1 Jin of Zhongru［钟乳, Stalactite, Stalactitum］and grind into powder. Prepare 3 Liang of Renshen［人参, Ginseng, Radix Ginseng］and remove the top. Prepare 5 Liang of Gancao［甘草, Liquorice Root, Glycyrrhiza uralensis Fisch］, roast them slightly brown and file into powder. Prepare 3 Liang of Gandihuang［干地黄, dried rehmannia, Rehmanniae Radix］. Prepare 2 Liang of Huangqi［黄芪, Milkvetch Root, Radix Astragali seu Hedysari］and file into powder. Prepare 3 Liang of Duzhong〔杜仲, eucommia, Eucommiae Cortex〕and remove the wrinkles. Prepare 6 Liang of Roucongrong〔肉苁蓉, Cistanche, Cistanches Herba〕. Prepare 5 Liang of Baifuling〔白茯苓, white poria, Poria Alba〕. Prepare 4 Liang of Maimendong〔麦门冬, Radix Ophiopogonis, Ophiopogon japonicus Ker-Gawl〕and remove the core part. Prepare 6 Liang of Shuyu〔薯蓣, Dioscorea, Dioscoreae Rhizoma〕. Prepare 2 Liang of Shihu〔石斛, dendrobe, Herba Dendrobii〕, romove its root and file into powder.

上药为末。以水三斗，先煮粟米七升为粥，放盆内。用药一两搅令匀，少和冷水，与渴牛饮之令足。不足更饮之一日。饮时患渴，不饮清水，平旦取牛乳服之，生熟任意。牛须三岁以上，七岁以下，纯黄色者为上，余色为下。其乳常令犊子饮之，若犊子不饮者，其乳动气，不堪服也。慎蒜、猪、鱼、生冷、陈、臭。其乳牛清洁养之，洗刷饮饲须如法，用心看之。

Grind the above ingredients into powder. Boil the millet in 3 Dou of water until 7 Sheng of porridge is left. Put it in a pot and add 1 Liang of the medicinal powder. Mix them well, add some cold water and feed the thirsty cow until it is full once a day. The cow can be fed with water other time in the day. Get the milk and drink it from 3:00 a.m. to 5:00 a.m. It does not matter if it is boiled or not. The cow should be 3 to 7 years old. Yellow cows are better than those in other colors. Let the calf drink the milk from the cow often. If the calf dislikes the milk, it may disorder qi and is not proper to take. Try not to eat garlic, pork, fish, raw and cold food, rotten and smelly food.

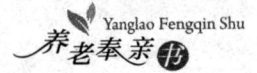

The cow should be kept in a clean environment and be cleaned and fed with great caution.

食治老人频遭重病，虚羸不可平复，宜服此。枸杞煎方。

Gouqi Jian（Decocted Barbary Wolfberry Fruit Formula）can be used to treat the aged who suffer from frequent sever diseases, persistent deficiency and emaciation.

生枸杞根细锉一斗，以水五斗，煮取一斗五升，澄清　白羊脊骨一具，锉碎

Take 1 Dou of fresh root of Gouqi ［枸杞, Barbary Wolfberry Fruit, Fructus Lycii］ and grind it with a file. Boil it in 5 Dou of water until 1.5 Dou of water is left and remove the dregs. Take a lamb spine and chop it into pieces.

上件药，以微火煎取五升，去滓，取入瓷合中。每服一合，与酒一少盏合暖，每于食前温服。

Decoct the above ingredients with slow fire until 5 Sheng is left, remove the dregs and put the decoction into porcelain bowl with lid. Warm 1 He of the decoction with a small cup of wine and take it before meals.

食治老人补五劳七伤虚损。法煮羊头方。

Fazhu Yangtou Fang（Boiled Sheep-head Formula）can be used to treat deficiency due to 5 kinds of consumptive diseases and 7 damages.

白羊头蹄一副，头蹄须用草火烧令黄色，刮去灰尘　胡椒半两　荜茇半两

干姜半两　葱白切半升　豉半斤

Prepare one white sheep head and a pair of sheep feet. Burn them brown with grass fire and remove the dust on the surface. Prepare 0.5 Liang of pepper, 0.5 Liang of Biji［荜茇, Long Pepper, Piper Longum L.］and dried ginger respectively. Prepare 0.5 Jin of chopped scallion and Douchi［豆豉, Fermented Soybean, Semen Sojae Preparatum］respectively.

上件药，先以水煮头蹄半熟，内药，更煮令烂，去骨，空腹适性食之。日食一具，满七具即止。禁生、冷、醋、滑、五辛、陈臭、猪、鸡等七日。

Boil the sheep head and feet until half-cooked. Put the above ingredients in water and cook it until it is ready. Remove the bone and take it with an empty stomach. Take one dose for one day and repeat it 7 days. It is contraindicated with anything raw or cold, vinegar, stimulating and greasy food, 5 kinds of food with pungent taste, food that is rotten and smelly, pork, and chicken.

治老人大虚羸困极，宜服。煎猪肪方。

Jian Zhufang Fang (Boiled Pork Lard Formula) is used to treat deficiency, emaciation and exhaustion of the aged.

猪肪不中水者半斤

Prepare 0.5 Jin of pork fat that is not contacted with water.

上，入葱白一茎于铛内，煎令葱黄即止。候冷暖如身体，空腹频服之令尽，暖盖覆卧。至日晡后，乃白粥调糜。过三日后，宜服羊肝羹。

Put the above ingredients and one piece of Chinese onion stalk into the stew-pan. Cook until the Chinese onion brown. Wait until it is of the body temperature. Take it in small portion frequently on an empty stomach and then lie with thick quilt covered to keep warm. Take some thoroughly cooked rice porridge after 5:00 p.m. It is advisable to have some sheep liver soup three days later.

羊肝羹方。

羊肝一具，去筋膜细切　羊脊肉二条，细切　曲末半两　枸杞根五斤，锉，以水一斗五升，煮取四升，去滓

Yanggan Geng Fang（Sheep Liver Soup Formula）.

Prepare one sheep liver, remove the membrane and slice thinly. Prepare 2 chunks of sheep filet and slice thinly. Prepare 5 Jin of root of Gouqi [枸杞, Barbary Wolfberry Fruit, Fructus Lycii], grind it with a slicer, boil it with 1.5 Dou of water until 4 Sheng of water is left, and remove the dregs.

上，用枸杞汁煮前羊肝等，令烂。入豉一小盏，葱白七茎切，以五味调和作羹，空腹饱食之。后三日，慎食如上法。

Boil the above ingredients with Gouqi soup until the sheep liver is tender. Put a small bowl of Douchi [豆豉, Fermented Soybean, Semen Sojae Preparatum] and 7 pieces of chopped scallion in and flavor them with 5 kinds of seasonings. Take it on an empty stomach and repeat taking this formula cautiously in the next 3 days.

食治老人，补虚劳。油面馎饦方。

Youmian Botuo Fang (Formula of Botuo① Served with Linseed Oil) is used to treat the aged with deficiency due to over-strain.

生胡麻油一斤　折粳米泔清一斤

Prepare 1 Jin of crude linseed oil and 1 Jin of washing water of polished rice.

上二味，以微火煎，尽泔清乃止，出贮之。取合盐汤二合，将和面作馎饦，煮令熟，入五味食之。

Boil the above 2 ingredients with slow fire until the water is clear enough. Remove from heat. Mix it with 2 He of salty water to make hand-pulled dough and cook it thoroughly. Take after flavor it with 5 kinds of seasonings.

增补方剂
Supplementary Formulas

《千金翼方》耆婆汤。主大虚冷风，羸弱，无颜色方。一云酥蜜汤。

The Qipo Decoction from *Qianjin Yifang* (*Supplement to Prescriptions Worth a Thousand Gold Pieces*): It is mainly used to treat severe deficiency, wind-cold, emaciation and pale complexion. It is also called Butter Honey

---

① Botuo: a cooked hand-pulled wheaten food.

Decoction.

酥一斤，炼　生姜一合，切　薤白三握，炙令黄　酒二升　白蜜一斤，炼　油一升　椒一合，汗　胡麻仁一升　橙叶一握，炙令黄　豉一升　糖一升

Prepare 1 Jin of butter and refine it. Prepare 1 He of chopped fresh ginger. Get 3 handful of Chinese chive and broil it to brown color. Prepare 2 Sheng of wine. Prepare 1 Jin of white honey and refine it. Prepare 1 Sheng of oil. Prepare 1 He of pepper and fry it slightly. Roast 1 Sheng of black sesame and a handful of orange leaves to brown. Prepare 1 Sheng of Douchi［豆豉，Fermented Soybean, Semen Sojae Preparatum］and 1 Sheng of sugar.

上一十一味，先以酒渍豉一宿，去滓，纳糖蜜油酥于铜器中，煮令匀沸。次纳薤姜，煮令熟。次下椒、橙叶、胡麻，煮沸。下二升豉汁，又煮一沸，出内瓷器中密封。空腹吞一合，如人行十里，更一服。冷者加椒。

（卷十二·养性·养老食疗第四）

Soak the above 11 ingredients in wine for one night and remove the dregs. Put the sugar, honey, oil and butter in copper ware and boil. Then put chive and ginger in the pot and cook them thoroughly. Then put the pepper, orange leaves, black sesame in the pot and boil. Then put 2 Sheng of fermented soya beans and boil. Take them out and seal in a porcelain pot. Take one He on an empty stomach. Take another dose in the time needed for walking 10 Li（about 3.1 miles）. Flavor with pepper if there is cold symptom.

（Volume 12 · *Self-cultivation· Chapter 4 Diet therapy for the Aged*）

邹氏三妙汤。实气养血，久服弥益人。

Zou's Decoction of Three Effective Ingredients: Replenish qi and nourish blood. Long-term taking of it benefits health.

地黄、枸杞实各取汁一升，蜜半升

Prepare 1 Sheng of Dihuang［地黄, Unprocessed Rehmannia Root, Rehmannia glutinosa Libosch. ex Fisch. et Mey.］juice and Gouqi［枸杞, Barbary Wolfberry Fruit, Fructus Lycii］juice separately and half Sheng of honey.

银器中同煎如稀饧。每服一大匕，汤调酒调皆可。

Boil them in silver ware till they are like maltose-like. Take one big spoon of it for one time. It can be taken together with soup or wine.

邹氏山芋粥。薯蓣生于山者名山药，一名山芋。山芋生山者佳，圃种者无味。取去皮，细石上磨如糊。每碗粥用山芋一合，以酥二合，蜜一合约炒令凝，以匙揉碎。粥欲熟，投搅令匀乃出。

（邹铉《寿亲养老新书》卷三）

The Yam gruel of Zou's: The Chinese yam grown in the mountains is called Shanyao in Chinese. It is also called Shanyu. The yam grown in the mountains is of high quality while those planted in the garden are not tasty. Peel and mash into paste on fine stone. To make one bowl of gruel, fry 1 He of yam, 2 He of butter and 1 He of honey to solid and mash it with a spoon.

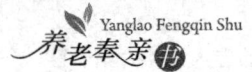

When the gruel is about to be cooked, put the mash in it and stir well.

（ Volume 3 of *The New Book for Keeping Longevity and Supporting Aged Relative*s by Zou Xuan ）

食治眼目方
Formulas to Treat Eye Diseases of the Aged with Diet Therapy

一

食治老人肝脏虚弱，远视，无力。补肝猪肝羹方。

I

Bugan Zhugan Geng Fang（Liver-Tonifying Pork Liver Soup Formula）is used to treat deficiency of the liver, farsightedness and fatigue of the aged.

猪肝一具，细切，去筋膜　葱白一握，去须切　鸡子二枚

Prepare one pig liver, slice thinly and remove the membrane. Take a handful of Chinese onion stalk and remove the root. Prepare 2 eggs.

上以豉汁中煮，作羹。临熟，打破鸡子，投在内食之。

Boil the above ingredients in fermented soybean juice. When it is about to be cooked, crack the eggs into the soup.

又方：

Another formula:

青羊肝一具，细切，水煮熟，漉干

Prepare one sheep liver and slice it thinly. Boil with water and then drain water off.

上以盐、酱、醋和食之立效。

Flavor with salt, sauce and vinegar and take. It is effective to cure the disease.

又方：

Another formula:

葱子半升，炒熟

Fry half Sheng of Chinese onion seeds.

上为末，每服一匙，以水二大盏，煎取一盏，去滓，入米，煮粥食之。

Grind them into powder. Take one spoon for one serving. Boil in 2 cups of water and decoct to 1 cup. Remove the dregs and make gruel with rice.

食治老人青白翳，明目，除邪气，利大肠，去寒热。马齿实拌葱豉粥方。

Machishi *Ban Congchi Zhou Fang*（Formula of Purslane Seed Mixed with Onion and Fermented Soy Beans）is used to treat eye screen of the aged. It can be used to brighten the eyes, expel pathogenic qi, disinhibit the large intestine, eliminate cold and heat.

马齿实一升

Prepare 1 Sheng of Machishi［马齿实, Purslane Seed, Portulacae Semen］.

上为末，每服一匙，煮葱豉粥，和搅食之。马齿菜作羹粥吃，并明目极佳。

Grind the above ingredient into powder. Take one spoon for one time, add Chinese onion and Douchi［豆豉, Fermented Soybean, Semen Sojae Preparatum］to make gruel. Stir well before serving.

食治老人肝脏风虚，眼暗。乌鸡肝粥方。

Wujigan Zhou Fang（Black-bone Chicken Liver Gruel Formula）is used to treat wind and deficiency of the liver and dim vision of the aged.

乌鸡肝一具，细切

Prepare one black-bone chicken liver and slice it thinly.

上以豉和米，作羹粥食之。

Mix the above ingredients with rice and Douchi［豆豉, Fermented Soybean, Semen Sojae Preparatum］to cook gruel.

食治老人目暗不明。苍耳粥方。

Cang'er Zhou Fang（Cang'erzi Gruel Formula）is used to treat dim vision of the aged.

苍耳子半两　粳米半升

The formula is composed of half Liang of Cang'erzi［苍耳子, Xanthium, Xanthii Fructus］, and half Sheng of polished round-grained rice.

上件，捣苍耳子烂。用布绞滤，以水一升，取汁和米煮粥食之。或作散，煎服亦佳。

Mash the Cang'erzi［苍耳子, Xanthium, Xanthii Fructus］and mix the above ingredients in 2 Sheng of water and filter with a piece of cloth. Cook gruel with rice. It is also effective to take in the form of powder or decoction.

二

食治老人热发，眼赤涩痛。栀子仁粥方。

II

Zhiziren Zhou Fang（Gardenia Seed Gruel Formula）is used to treat fever, pain and redness of the eyes of the aged.

栀子仁一两

Prepare 1 Liang of Zhiziren［栀子仁, Gardenia Seed, Gardeniae Semen］.

上为末，分为四服。每服用米三合煮粥，临熟时下栀子末一分，搅令匀食之。

Grind the above ingredients into powder and divide to 4 servings. Make gruel with 3 He of rice for each dose, when it is almost ready, add 1 Fen of gardenia powder. Mix it well and eat.

食治老人益精气，强志意，聪耳目。鸡头实粥方。

Jitoushi Zhou Fang（Gordon Euryale Seed Gruel Formula）is used to boost essence, enhance will power, sharpen hearing and brighten the eyes.

鸡头实三合

Prepare 3 He of Jitoushi ［鸡头实, Gordon Euryale Seed, Semen Euryales］.

上，煮令熟，去壳，研如膏。入粳米一合，煮粥，空腹食。

Boil thoroughly, remove the hull and grind to paste. Cook gruel with 1 He of polished round-grained rice and take on an empty stomach.

治老人补中明目，利小便。蔓菁粥方。

Manjing Zhou Fang（Turnip Seed Gruel Formula）is used to tonify the center, brighten the eyes and disinhibit urine.

蔓菁子二合　粳米三合

It is composed of 2 He of Manjingzi ［蔓菁子, Turnip Seed, Brassicae Rapae Semen］ and 3 He of polished round-grained rice.

上捣碎，入水二大盏，绞滤取汁，著米煮粥空心食之。

Mash the above ingredients and then soak it in 2 big cups of water, squeeze and filter to get the juice. Cook gruel with the juice and take on an empty stomach.

食治老人益耳目聪明，补中强志。莲实粥方。

Lianshi Zhou Fang（Lotus Fruit Gruel Formula）is used to sharpen hearing and vision, tonify the center and keep up the spirit of the aged.

莲实半两，去皮，细切　糯米三合

It is composed of half Liang of Lianshi［莲实, Lotus Fruit, Nelumbinis Semen］sliced thinly with the skin removed and 3 He of glutinous rice.

上，先以水煮莲实令熟，次入糯米作粥，候熟，入莲实搅令匀，热食之。

Boil Lianshi［莲实, Lotus Fruit, Nelumbinis Semen］thoroughly and filter it out. Then add glutinous rice to make gruel. When it is cooked, add Lianshi［莲实, Lotus Fruit, Nelumbinis Semen］and stir well. Take while it is hot.

食治老人膈上风热、头目赤痛、目视䀮䀮。竹叶粥方。

Zhuye Zhou Fang（Bamboo Leaves Gruel Formula）is used to treat wind-heat in the diaphragm, pain and redness of the eyes and head, and dim vision of the aged.

竹叶五十片,净洗　石膏三两　砂糖一两　折粳米三合

It is composed of 50 clean Bamboo leaves, 3 Liang of Shigao [石膏, Gypsum, Gypsum Fibrosum], 1 Liang of granulated sugar, and 3 He of polished round-grained rice.

上以水三大盏，煎石膏等二味，取二盏。去滓澄清，用煮粥熟，入砂糖食之。

Boil the above ingredients in 3 big cups of water and decoct with Shigao [石膏, Gypsum, Gypsum Fibrosum] to 2 cups remains. Remove the dregs and make gruel. Flavor it with sugar.

增补方剂
Supplementary Formulas

《备急千金要方》补肝散。治失明漠漠方。

Liver-supplementing powder in *Beiji Qianjin Yaofang* (*Valuable Prescriptions For Emergency*) is used to treat loss of sight.

青羊肝一具，去上膜薄切之，以新瓦瓶子未用者，净拭之，内肝于中，炭火上炙之令极干，汁尽，末之　决明子半升　蓼子一合，熬令香

Prepare 1 goat liver, remove the membrane and cut it thinly. Put it in a new earthen jar and roast on fire to dry it, then grind it into powder. Prepare half Sheng of Juemingzi [决明子, Seed of Sickle Senna, Semen Cassiae]. Boil 1 He of Liaozi [蓼子, Slender Bearded Smartweed, Polygoni Gracilis Herba et Radix] throughly.

上三昧合治，下筛。以粥饮，食后服方寸匕，日二，稍加至三匕，不过两剂。能一岁服之，可夜读细书。

Mix the above ingredients and sieve. Take as the gruel after meal. One square-inch-spoon for a serving, twice a day, or take 3 square-inch-spoon for a serving and no more than 2 servings a day. After one-year taking, one can read small print at night.

食治耳聋耳鸣诸方
Formulas to Treat Deaf and Tinnitus of the Aged with Diet Therapy

一

食治老人久患耳聋，养肾脏，强骨气。磁石猪肾羹方。

I

Cishi Zhushen Geng Fang（Loadstone Pig Kidney Soup Formula）is used to treat long-term deafness, nourish the kidney and strengthen the bone of the aged.

磁石一斤，杵碎，水淘去赤，用绵裹　猪肾一对，去脂膜，细切

Prepare 1 Jin of Cishi［磁石, Loadstone, Magnetitum］, and smash with a pestle. Elutriate with water to remove the red impurity, and put it in a piece of cotton gauze. Prepare 2 pig kidneys, remove the membrane and slice thinly.

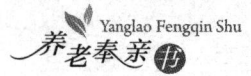

上，以水五升，煮磁石，取二升。去磁石，投肾调和。以葱豉、姜、椒作羹，空腹食之。作粥及入酒并得。磁石常留起，依前法用之。

Boil the above ingredients in 5 Sheng of water until 2 Sheng remains. Take out the Cishi ［磁石, Loadstone, Magnetitum］ and add pig kidneys. Cook soup with Chinese onion, Douchi ［豆豉, Fermented Soybean, Semen Sojae Preparatum］, ginger, and pepper. Take on an empty stomach. It is effective to take as gruel or mix with wine. Put the Cishi ［磁石, Loadstone, Magnetitum］ away and use next time as usual.

食治老人肾气虚损，耳聋。鹿肾粥方。

Lushen Zhou Fang（Deer Kidney Gruel Formula）is used to treat deficiency of kidney qi and deafness of the aged.

鹿肾一对，去脂膜，切　　粳米三合

Prepare 2 deer kidneys, remove the membrane and chop it into pieces. Prepare 3 He of polished round-grained rice.

上，于豉汁中相和，煮作粥。入五味，如法调和，空腹食之。作羹及作酒并得。

Mix the above ingredients with Douchi ［豆豉, Fermented Soybean, Semen Sojae Preparatum］ juice and make gruel. Flavor with 5 kinds of seasonings and take on an empty stomach. It is effective to take as gruel or mix with wine.

二

食治老人五脏气壅，耳聋。乌鸡膏粥方。

II

Wujigao Zhou Fang（Black-bone Chicken Fat Gruel Formula）is used to treat deafness due to qi stagnation of the five zang-organs.

乌鸡脂一两　粳米三合

It is composed of 1 Liang of black-bone chicken fat and 3 He of polished round-grained rice.

上相和，煮粥。入五味调和，空腹食之。乌鸡脂和酒饮，亦佳。

Make gruel with the above ingredients. Season with 5 kinds of seasonings and take on an empty stomach. It is also good to take with wine.

食治老人耳聋不差。鲤鱼脑髓粥方。

Liyu Naosui Zhou Fang（Carp Brain Gruel Formula）is used to treat long-term deafness of the aged.

鲤鱼脑髓二两　粳米三合

It is composed of 2 Liang of carp brain and 3 He of polished round-grained rice.

上，煮粥。以五味调和，空腹服之。

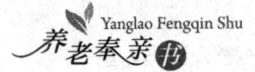

Make gruel with the above ingredients. Season with 5 kinds of seasonings and take on an empty stomach.

食治老人肾脏气惫，耳聋。猪肾粥方。

Zhushen Zhou Fang（Pig Kidney gruel Formula）is used to treat exhaustion in the kidney and deafness of the aged.

猪肾一两，去膜，细切　葱白二茎，去须切　人参一分，去芦头　防风一分，去芦　粳米二合　薤白去茎，去须

Prepare 2 pig kidneys, remove membrane and slice thinly. Take 2 pieces of scallion, remove the root and slice. Prepare 1 Fen of Renshen〔人参，Ginseng, Radix Ginseng〕with the top removed, and 1 Fen of Fangfeng〔防风，Divaricate Saposhnikovia Root, Radix Saposhnikoviae〕with the top removed. Prepare 2 He of polished round-grained rice. Prepare Xiebai〔薤白，Chinese chive, Allii Macrostemonis Bulbus〕with the stem and roots removed.

上件药末，并米、葱、薤白，著水下锅中。煮候粥临熟，拨开中心，下肾，莫搅动，慢火更煮良久，入五味，空腹服之。

Grind the above ingredients into powder. Add rice, Chinese onion, Xiebai〔薤白 Chinese chive, Allii Macrostemonis Bulbus〕to the the water. When the gruel is about to be cooked, put the kidneys into the center without stiring, simmer for a fairly long time. Flavor with 5 kinds of seasonings and take on an empty stomach.

增补方剂

Supplementary Formulas

《太平圣惠方》治耳聋，及不闻香臭。干柿粥方。

According to *Taiping Shenghui Fang*（*Taiping Holy Preions for Universal Relief*）, Dried persimmon gruel formula can be used to treat deafness and nasal congestion inhibiting the sense of smell.

干柿三枚，细切　粳米三合

Slice 3 dried Shi ［柿, Persimmon, Kaki Fructus Exsiccatus］ thinly and prepare 3 He of polished round-grained rice.

上，于豉汁中煮粥，空腹食之。

Make gruel with the above ingredients in Douchi ［豆豉, Fermented Soybean, Semen Sojae Preparatum］ juice. Take on an empty stomach.

食治五劳七伤诸方

Formulas to Treat Five Kinds of Consumptive Diseases and Seven Damages of the Aged with Diet Therapy

食治老人五劳七伤，下焦虚冷，小便遗精，宜食。暖腰壮阳道饼子方。

Nuanyao Zhuangyangdao Bingzi Fang（Waist-warming and Yang-invigorating Medicinal Cake Formula）is used to treat 5 kinds of consumptive diseases and 7 damages of the aged. It is suitable for the aged with lower burner insufficiency-cold and spermatorrhea.

附子一两，炮制，去皮脐　　神面曲三两　　干姜一两，炮制，锉　　桂心一两　　五味子一两　　肉苁蓉一两半，酒浸一宿，刮去皱皮，炙干　　菟丝子一两，酒浸三日，曝干为末　　羊髓二两　　大枣二十枚，煮，去皮核　　酥二两　　蜜四两　　白面一斤　　黄牛乳一斤半　　汉椒半两，去目及闭口者，微炒，去汗

Process 1 Liang of Fuzi ［附子, Aconite, Radix Aconiti Praeparata］ processed with the skin and navel removed. Prepare 3 Liang of Shenqu ［神曲, Medicated Leaven, Massa Medicata Fermentata］, 1 Liang of dried gingerprocessed and filed, 1 Liang of Guixin ［桂心, Cinnamon Bark, Cortex Cinnamomi］, 1 Liang of Wuweizi ［五味子, Chinese Magnoliavine Fruit, Fructus Schisandrae Chinensis］, and 2 Liang of lamb bone marrow. Boil twenty Chinese dates with the skin and core removed. Prepare 2 Liang of butter, 4 Liang of honey, 1 Jin of flour and 1.5 Jin of milk. Steep 1.5 Liang of Roucongrong ［肉苁蓉, Cistanche, Cistanches Herba］ in wine for a night and then remove the skin. Steep 1 Liang of Tusizi ［菟丝子, Cuscuta, Cuscutae Semen］ into wine for 3 days, dry in the sun to make powder. Prepare half Liang of Sichuan pepper. Pick out those whose skin does not crack. Stir for a while to remove the water.

上为末。入面，以酥、蜜、髓、乳相和，入枣瓤熟，搜于盘中，盖覆，勿令通风，半日久即将出。更搜令熟，擀作糊饼大，面上以筋挑之。即入炉中，上下以火煿令熟。每日空腹食五枚。一方入酵和更佳。

Grind the above ingredients into powder. Mix it with flour, butter, honey, marrow and milk. Add pitted Chinese dates and cook thoroughly. Put it on a plate and cover for half a day to make sure there is no expose to air. Roll it into cakes and fry it in a griddle. Take 5 cakes on an empty stomach every day. According to another formula, fermentation will make it better.

食治老人五劳七伤，益下元，壮气海。服经月余，肌肉充盛。老成少年，并宜服食。雌鸡粥方。

Ciji Zhou Fang（Hen Gruel Formula）is used to treat 5 kinds of consumptive diseases and 7 damages of the aged. It can boost lower origin and strengthen sea of qi. Taking for more than a month will strengthen the muscle. It is effective for all ages.

黄雌鸡一只，去毛、脏腹　肉苁蓉酒浸一宿，一两，刮去皱皮，切　生薯蓣一两，切　阿魏少许，炼过　粳米二合，淘入

Prepare 1 yellow hen. Pluck the feathers and remove the inner organs. Prepare 1 Liang of Shengshuyu［生薯蓣, Raw Dioscorea, Dioscoreae Rhizoma Crudum］and slice. A little A'wei［阿魏, Asafetida, Ferulae Resina］fried. Wash 1 He of polished round-grained rice and add into the wok. Steep 1 Liang of Roucongrong［肉苁蓉, Cistanche, Cistanches Herba］in wine for 1 night, remove the wrinkled skin and slice.

以上，先将鸡烂煮，擘骨取汁，下米及鸡、肉苁蓉等，都煮粥。入五味，空心食之。

Boil the chicken until it is cooked. Break off the bones, put the other ingredients in. Flavor with 5 kinds of seasonings and take on an empty stomach.

食治五劳七伤，阳气衰弱，腰脚无力，宜食。羊肾苁蓉羹方。

Yangshen Congrong Geng Fang（Soup Formula of Lamb Kidney and Cistanche）is used to treat 5 kinds of consumptive diseases and 7 damages, weak yang qi, weak waist and legs of the aged.

羊肾一对，去筋、膜、脂，细切　肉苁蓉一两，酒浸二宿，刮去皱皮，细切

Prepare 2 lamb kidneys, remove the membrane and fat, slice thinly. Steep 1 Liang of Roucongrong［肉苁蓉, Cistanche, Cistanches Herba］in wine for 2 nights, remove the wrinkled skin and slice thinly.

上件药，和作羹。著葱白、盐、五味末等，一如常法。空腹服之。

Cook gruel with the above ingredients. Add Chinese onion stalk, salt, 5-ingredient powder as usual. Take on an empty stomach.

二

食治老人五劳七伤，阳气衰弱，强益气力。鹿肾粥方。

II

Lushen Zhou Fang（Deer Kidney Gruel Formula）is used to treat 5 kinds of consumptive diseases and 7 damages, yang debilitation, replenish qi and strength of the aged.

鹿肾一对，去脂膜细切　肉苁蓉二两，酒浸一宿，刮去皮，切　粳米三合

Prepare 2 deer kidneys, remove the membrane and slice thinly. Steep 2 Liang of Roucongrong ［肉苁蓉, Cistanche, Cistanches Herba］ in wine for 1 night, remove the skin and slice. Prepare 2 He of polished round-grained rice.

上件药，先以水二盏，煮米作粥，欲熟，下鹿肾、苁蓉、葱。

Boil the above ingredients in 2 cups of water, when it is about to be cooked, add deer kidneys, Roucongrong ［肉苁蓉, Cistanche, Cistanches Herba］ and Chinese onion.

增补方剂
Supplementary Formulas

《圣惠方》治五劳七伤，庶事衰弱。枸杞粥方。

It is recorded in *Taiping Shenghui Fang* (*Taiping Holy Prescriptions for Universal Relief*) that Wolf-berry gruel formula can treat 5 kinds of consumptive diseases and 7 damages, and debility.

枸杞菜半斤切　粳米二合

It is composed of half Jin of sliced Gouqicai ［枸杞菜, Barbary Wolfberry Fruit, Fructus Lycii］ and 2 He of polished round-grained rice.

上件，以豉汁相和，煮作粥。以五味葱白等，调和食之。

Mix the above ingredients in Douchi 〔豆豉, Fermented Soybean, Semen Sojae Preparatum〕 juice to cook gruel. Flavor with 5 kinds of seasonings, Chinese onion stalk, etc. before serving.

《太平圣惠方》治五劳七伤，阴囊下湿痒。萝藦菜粥方。

It is recorded in *Taiping Shenghui Fang*（*Taiping Holy Prescriptions for Universal Relief*）that Metaplexis Japonica gruel formula can be used to treat scrotal damp itch.

萝藦菜半斤　羊肾一对，去脂膜　粳米二合

It is composed of half Jin of Luomo 〔萝藦, Metaplexis Japonica, Metaplexis Japonica Makino〕, 2 lamb kidneys with the membrane removed, and 2 He of polished round-grained rice.

上细切煮粥，调和如常法，空腹食之。

Slice the above ingredients thinly, flavor as usual and take on an empty stomach.

《太平圣惠方》治五劳七伤，阴痿气弱。鸡肝粥方。

It is recorded in *Taiping Shenghui Fang*（*Taiping Holy Prescriptions for Universal Relief*）that chicken liver gruel can treat 5 kinds of consumptive diseases, 7 damages, impotence and weak qi.

雄鸡肝一具，切　菟丝子末半两　粟米二合

Prepare one cock liver, half Liang Tusizi〔菟丝子, Cuscuta, Cuscutae Semen〕powder, 2 He of millet.

上以水二大盏半,入五味及葱,煮作粥,空心食之。

Boil the above ingredients in 2.5 big cups of water, add 5 kinds of seasonings and Chinese onion to cook gruel. Take on an empty stomach.

(以上三方摘自卷九十七,食治五劳七伤诸方)

(The above formulas are selected from Volume 97: *Formulas to Treat Five Kinds of Consumptive Diseases and Seven Damages.*)

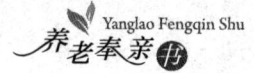

食治虚损羸瘦诸方

Formulas to Treat Deficiency and Emaciation of the Aged with Diet Therapy

食治老人脏腑虚损，羸瘦，阳气乏弱。雀儿粥方。

Que'er Zhou Fang (Sparrow Gruel Formula) is used to treat deficiency of zang-fu organs, emaciation, insufficiency yang qi of the aged.

雀儿五只，治如食法，细切 粟米一合 葱白三茎，切

Prepare 5 sparrows as the usual way before serving and slice thinly. Prepare 1 He of millet. Take 3 pieces of scallions and slice.

上先将雀儿炒肉，次入酒一合，煮少时，入水二大盏半，下米煮作粥，欲熟，下葱白、五味等。候熟，空心服之。

Fry the sparrows first, and then add 1 He of wine. Boil for a while and add 2.5 big cups of water. Cook gruel with the millet. When it is about to be boiled, add scallions and 5 kinds of seasonings. When it is well boiled, take on an empty stomach.

食治老人虚损羸瘦，下焦久冷，眼昏耳聋。骨汁煮饼方。

Guzhi Zhubing Fang (Formula of Noodles Cooked in Bone Soup) is used to treat deficiency, emaciation, enduring cold in lower energizer, dim vision and deafness of the aged.

大羊尾骨一条，以水五大盏，煮取汁二大盏五分　　葱白五茎，去须，切　　面三两　　陈橘皮一两，汤浸去白瓤，焙　　羊肉四两，细切　　荆芥一握

Boil a big lamb tail bone with 5 big cups of water until 2.5 cups of soup is left. Take 5 pieces of scallions, remove the root and slice. Prepare 1 Liang of Chenjupi〔陈皮, Dried Tangerine Peel, Pericarpium Citri Reticulatae〕, wash to remove the pith, then bake. Prepare a handful of Jingjie〔荆芥, Fineleaf Schizonepeta Herb, Herba Schizonepetae〕, 3 Liang of flour, and 4 Liang of thinly-sliced lamb.

上件药，都用骨汁煮五七沸，去滓。用汁少许后，搜面作索饼，却于汁中与羊肉煮，入五味，空腹服之。

Boil the above ingredients in bone soup for a while and remove the dregs. Make noodles with a little soup and ferment flour. Put the noodles into the pot to cook with the lamb. Flavor with 5 kinds of seasonings and take on an empty stomach.

食治老人虚损羸瘦，助阳壮筋骨。羊肉粥方。

Yangrou Zhou Fang（Lamb Gruel Formula）is used to treat deficiency, emaciation, assisting yang and strengthting sinew and bones of the aged.

羊肉二斤　　黄芪一两，生锉　　人参一两，去芦头　　白茯苓一两　　枣五枚　　粳米三合

Prepare 2 Jin of lamb, file 1 Liang of Huangqi〔黄芪, Milkvetch Root, Radix Astragali seu Hedysari〕. Prepare 1 Liang of Renshen〔人参, Ginseng,

Radix Ginseng] and remove the top. Prepare 1 Liang of Baifuling [white poria, Poria Alba], 5 Chinese dates and 3 He of polished round-grained rice.

上件药，先将肉去脂皮，取精膂肉，留四两细切，余一斤十二两，以水五大盏，并黄芪等，煎取汁三盏，去滓。入米煮粥，临熟，下切了生肉，更煮。入五味调和，空心食之。

Remove the fat and skin, and keep the lean meat. Get 4 Liang of it sliced thinly. Boil the rest lean meat in 5 big cups of water with Huangqi [黄芪, Milkvetch Root, Radix Astragali seu Hedysari] and the other ingredients. Cook until 3 cups of decoction remains and then remove the dregs. Add rice to cook gruel. Add the lean meat when it is about to be cooked, and boil it for a while. Flavor with 5 kinds of seasonings and take on an empty stomach.

食治老人虚损羸瘦，令人肥白光泽。鸡子索饼方。

Jizi Suobing Fang (Egg Noodle Formula) is used to treat deficiency, emaciation of the aged, to make them have glow skin.

白面四两　鸡子四两　白羊肉四两，炒作臛

It is composed of 4 Liang of flour, 4 Liang of eggs and 4 Liang of thinly-sliced lamb fried into broth.

上件，以鸡子清搜面作索饼，于豉汁中煮令熟。入五味和臛，空腹食之。

Use the above ingredients to make noodles, boil in the Douchi [豆豉, Fermented Soybean, Semen Sojae Preparatum] juice. Add broth and 5 kinds of seasonings, take on an empty stomach.

食治老人肾气损，阴痿，固痹，风湿肢节中痛，不可持物。石英水煮粥方。

Shiyingshui Zhuzhou Fang (White Quartz Gruel Formula) is used to treat deficiency of kidney qi, impotence, generalized impediment, pain in the limbs due to wind-damp and difficulty in grasping objects.

白石英二十两　磁石三十两，并捶碎

It is composed of 20 Liang of Baishiying [白石英, White Quartz, Description] and 30 Liang of Cishi [磁石, Loadstone, Magnetitum] smashed into powder.

上件药，以水二斗，器中浸，于露地安置。夜即揭盖，令得星月气。每日取水作羹粥及煎茶汤吃，皆用之。用却一升，即添一升。如此经年，诸风并差，气力强盛，颜如童子。

Soak the above ingredients in 2 Dou of water in the pot, and put it in the open air. Remove the lid at night to make it obtain qi from the moon and stars. Use the water to make gruel, tea, and soup every day. Add water after use. After long-term taking, disorders due to wind will be treated. Qi and strength will be exuberant, and the aged will look younger.

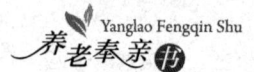

增补方剂
Supplementary Formulas

《太平圣惠方》治五脏虚损，羸瘦，益气力，坚筋骨。苣胜粥方。

According to *Taiping Shenghui Fang* (*Taiping Holy Prescriptions for Universal Relief*), Lettuce gruel formula can be used to treat deficiency of the five zang-organs, emaciation. It can replenish qi, strengthen sinews and bones.

苣胜子不限多少，拣去杂，蒸曝各九遍

Separate impurities from lettuce seeds, steam and put them under the blazing sun for 9 times.

上每取二合，用汤浸布裹，挼去皮，再研，水滤取汁，煎成饮，著粳米作粥食之。或煎浓饮，浇索饼食之，甚佳。

（摘自卷九十七·食治虚损羸瘦诸方）

Take 2 He of the above processed lettuce seeds, wrap with wet cloth, rub to remove the skin. Pestle and filter to get the extract, decoct with polished round-grained rice to make gruel. It is also effective to be decocted thickly and poured on the noodles.

（Volume 97 · *Formulas to Treat Deficiency and Emaciation of the Aged with Diet Therapy*）

食治脾胃气弱方

Formulas to Treat Qi Deficiency of the Spleen and the Stomach of the Aged with Diet Therapy

食治老人脾胃气弱，不多食，四肢困乏无力，黄瘦。羊肉索饼方。

Yangrou Suobing Fang（Lamb Noodles Formula）is used treat weak qi of the spleen and the stomach, poor appetite, fatigued limbs and yellowish complexion of the aged.

白羊肉四两　白面六两　生姜汁一合

It is composed of 4 Liang of lamb, 6 Liang of flour, and 1 He of ginger juice.

上，以姜汁搜面，肉切作臛头。下五味、椒、葱煮熟，空心食之，日一服，如常作益佳。

Mix the flour with ginger juice to make noodles, and slice the meat as condiment. Flavor with 5 kinds of seasonings, pepper and Chinese onion, cook them thoroughly. Take on an empty stomach once a day. Regular taking of it will be effective.

二

食治老人脾胃气弱，食饮不下，虚劣羸瘦，及气力衰微，行履不得。鲫鱼熟鲙方。

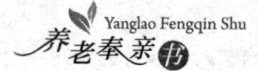

II

Jiyu Shukuai Fang (Sliced Crucian Carp Formula) is used to treat weak qi of the spleen and the stomach, indigestion, weakness, emaciation, fatigue, lack of strength and inability to walk.

鲫鱼肉半斤，细作鲙

Prepare half Jin of crucian carp and slice it thinly.

上，投豉汁中煮，令熟。下胡椒、莳萝并姜、橘皮等末及五味，空腹食。食常尤佳。

Boil the above ingredients in Douchi [豆豉, Fermented Soybean, Semen Sojae Preparatum] juice and cook thoroughly. Flavor with pepper, dill, ginger, tangerine peel and 5 kinds of seasonings. Take on an empty stomach. Long-term taking is good for health.

食治老人脾胃气弱，饮食不多，赢乏。藿菜羹方。

Huocai Geng Fang (Bean Seedling Gruel Formula) is used treat weak qi of the spleen and the stomach, poor appetite, emaciation, fatigue and lack of strength.

藿菜四两，切之　鲫鱼肉五两

Slice 4 Liang of bean seedlings and prepare 5 Liang of crucian carp.

上，煮作羹，下五味、椒、姜，并调少面，空心食之。常以三五日服，极补益。

Cook the above ingredients, add 5 kinds of seasonings, pepper and ginger, mix with a bit of flour. Take on an empty stomach. Take once every 3 to 5 days.

食治老人脾胃气弱，不能饮食，多困无力。酿猪肚方。
Niang Zhudu Fang（Brewed Pork Tripe Formula）is used treat weak qi of the spleen and stomach, inability to eat, tiredness and fatigue.

猪肚一个，肥者，净洗之　人参末半两　橘皮末半两　猪脾二枚，细切　饭半碗　葱白半握

The formula is composed of one clean fatty pork tripe, half Liang of Renshen［人参，Ginseng, Radix Ginseng］powder, half Liang of Jupi［橘皮，Tangerine Peel, Citri Reticulatae Pericarpium］powder, 2 thinly-sliced pork spleens, half bowl of rice and half a handful of scallion.

上，总内猪肚中相和，以椒、酱、五味讫，缝口合蒸之，令烂熟，空心渐食之。能作三两剂，兼补劳。

Stuff the pork tripe with the above ingredients, add pepper, sauce, and 5 kinds of seasonings. Then sew on the opening and steam it thoroughly. Take it slowly on an empty stomach. It is enough to make 2 or 3 doses. It can also be used to treat consumptive diseases.

食治老人脾胃气弱，不多进食，行步无力，黄瘦气微，见食即欲吐。

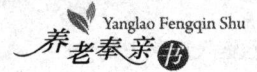

鸡子馎饦方。

Jizi Botuo Fang (Egg Hand-pulled Dough Soup Formula) is used to treat qi deficiency in the spleen and stomach, poor appetite, flaccidity, emaciation, shortness of breath and vomiting upon seeing food of the aged.

鸡子三枚　白面五两　白羊肉五两，作腥头

The formula is composed of 3 eggs, 5 Liang of flour, and 5 Liang of lamb as condiment.

上件，以鸡子白搜面，如常法作之。以五味煮熟，空心食之，日一服。常作极补虚。

Make long noodles with egg white as usual. Add 5 kinds of seasonings and cook thoroughly, Long-term taking will tonify deficiency.

食治老人脾胃气弱，食不消化，羸瘦，举动无力，多卧。曲末索饼子方。

Qumo Suobingzi Fang (Medicated Leaven Powder Noodle Formula) is used to treat weak qi of the spleen and stomach, non-transformation of food, emaciation, lack of strength, bedridden.

曲末二两，捣为面　白面五两　生姜汁三两　白羊肉二两，作腥头

Prepare 2 Liang of Shenqu [神曲, Medicated Leaven, Massa Medicata Fermentata] and grind it into powder. Prepare 5 Liang of flour, 3 He of ginger juice, and 2 Liang of lamb as condiment.

上以姜汁搜曲末和面作之，加羊肉臐头，及下酱、椒、五味，煮熟。空心食之。日一服。常服尤益。

Mix the flour with ginger juice and mutton condiment. Flavor with 5 kinds of seasonings and boil. Take on an empty stomach once a day. Long-term taking is good for health.

食治老人脾胃气弱，劳损，不下食。羊脊骨粥方。

Yangjirou Zhou Fang（Lamb Backbone Gruel Formula）is used to treat weak qi of the spleen and stomach, over-strain, and inability to take food of the aged.

大羊脊骨一具，肥者，捶碎　青粱米四合，净淘

It is composed of 1 fat mashed lamb spine and 4 He of clean Qingliangmi［青粱米, Seed of Foxtail Millet, Setaria italica］.

以上，水五升，煎取二升汁，下米煮作粥，空心食之。可下五味常服，其功难及，甚效。

Boil them in 5 Sheng of water until 2 Sheng of decoction remains. Add rice to make gruel and take on an empty stomach. It is very effective to take regularly flavored with 5 kinds of seasonings.

食治老人脾胃气弱，干呕，不能下食。羊血方。

Yangxue Fang（Lamb Blood Formula）is used to treat weak qi of the

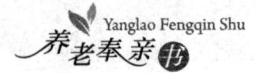

spleen and stomach, vomiting and inability to take food of the aged.

羊血一斤，鲜者，面酱作片　葱白一握　白面四两，捍切

Cut 1 Jin of fresh lamb blood into slices. Prepare a handful of Chinese onion stalk. Make dough with 4 Liang of flour, roll it and then slice to pieces.

上，煮血令熟，渐食之。三五服极有验，能补益脏腑。

Boil the above ingredients to make lamb blood cooked, and take gradually. Take 3 to 5 doses and it will take effect to tonify the zang-fu organs.

食治老人脾胃虚弱，呕吐，不下食，渐加羸瘦。粟米粥方。

Sumi Zhou Fang（Millet Gruel Formula）is used treat weak qi of the spleen and the stomach, vomiting, inability to take food and emaciation of the aged.

粟米四合，净淘　白面四两

The formula is composed of 4 He of millet and 4 Liang of flour. Wash the millet clean.

上，以粟米杵面令匀。煮作粥，空心食之，一日一服。极养肾气和胃。

Pound the above ingredients and stir well to make gruel. Take it on an empty stomach once a day. It is very effective to tonify the kidney qi and the stomach.

食治老人饮食不下，或呕逆虚弱。生姜汤方。

Shengjiang Tang Fang (Fresh Ginger Decoction Formula) is used to treat the poor appetite, vomiting, reverse flow of qi, and weakness of the aged.

生姜二两，去皮，细切　浆水一升

It is composed of 2 Liang of fresh ginger and 1 Sheng of sour millet water. Peel the fresh ginger and slice thinly.

上，和少盐，煎取七合，空心常作开胃进食。

Boil the above ingredients with a pinch of salt until 7 He of the liquid remains. Take on an empty stomach. Regular taking will increase the appetite and food intake.

食治老人脾胃虚弱，恶心，不欲饮食，常呕吐。虎肉炙方。

Hurou Zhi Fang (Roast Tiger Formula) is used treat weakness of the spleen and stomach, nausea, poor appetite, and frequent vomiting of the aged.

虎肉半斤，切，作胾　葱白半握，细切

Prepare half Jin of tiger meat and half a handful of scallion. Slice them thinly.

上件，以椒、酱、五味调，炙之。空心食，冷为佳。不可热食，损齿。

Add pepper, sauce and 5 kinds of seasonings to the above ingredients and roast. Take it cold on an empty stomach. Do not take it while it is still hot for it may damage the teeth.

食治老人脾胃气弱，不多食，痿瘦。黄雌鸡馄饨方。

Huangciji Huntun Fang（Yellow Hen Huntun Formula）is used treat weak qi of the spleen and stomach, poor appetite, and emaciation of the aged.

黄雌鸡肉五两　　白面七两　　葱白二合，细切

It is composed of 5 Liang of yellow hen, 7 Liang of flour and 2 He of thinly-sliced scallion.

上，以切肉作馄饨，下椒、酱、五味调和煮熟，空心食之，日一服。皆益脏腑，悦泽颜色。

Make Huntun with the above ingredients. Flavor with pepper, sauce, and 5 kinds of seasonings and cook thoroughly. Take on an empty stomach once a day. It can be used to tonify the zang-fu organs and refine complexion.

增补方剂
Supplementary Formulas

《寿亲养老新书》造山药面法：

The method to make Yam Flour is recorded in *Shouqin Yanglao Xinshu*

(*A New Book for Prolonging the Life-span of the Aged*).

取山药去皮薄切，日中暴干，柳箕中挼为粉，下筛。如常面食之，加酥蜜为 溲面尤精。益气力，长肌肉，久服轻身，耳目聪明，不饥延年。

Peel yam and slice thinly. Dry in the sun. Grind it into powder in winnowing basket and put it through a seive. Take it as wheaten food. It is more effective to add butter and honey to make noodles. It can be used to replenish qi and strength, engender muscles. Long-term taking of it will relax the body, improve vision and hearing, makes people feel less hungry, and enjoy a long lifespan.

《寿亲养老新书》人参粥：

The method to make Ginseng Gruel is recorded in *Shouqin Yanglao Xinshu* (*A New Book for Prolonging the Life-span of the Aged*).

人参半两，为末　生姜半两，取汁

Prepare half Liang of ginseng and grind it into powder. Extract juice from half Liang of fresh ginger.

上二味，以水一升，煮取一升。入粟米一合，煮为稀粥，觉饥即食之。治反胃，吐酸水。

Boil the above ingredients in 1 Sheng of water until 1 Sheng of soup remains. Add one He of millet to make gruel, and take when hungry. It can be used to treat gastric disorder causing nausea and acid-vomiting.

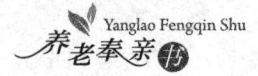

食治泻痢诸方
Formulas to Treat Diarrhea of the Aged with Diet Therapy

一

食治老人脾胃气冷，痢白脓涕，腰脊疼痛，瘦弱无力。鲫鱼熟鲙。

I

Jiyu Shukuai（Sliced Crucian Carp Formula）is used treat weak qi of the spleen and stomach, white dysentery and nasal mucus with pus, pain in lumbar spine and emaciation of the aged.

鲫鱼肉九两，切作鲙　豉汁七合　干姜半两　橘皮末半两

It is composed of 9 Liang of thinly-sliced crucian carp, 7 He of Douchi〔豆豉, Fermented Soybean, Semen Sojae Preparatum〕juice, half Liang of dried ginger, and half Liang of tangerine peel powder.

上以椒、酱、五味调和豉汁。沸即下鱼鲙煮熟，下二味，空心食之。日一服，其效尤益。

Add pepper, sauce, 5 kinds of seasonings and fermented soya beans juice to the above ingredients. Add crucian carp to the boiled soup, then put the other 2 ingredients in. Take on an empty stomach. It will be very effective to take once a day.

食治老人肠胃冷气，痢下不止。赤石脂馎饦方。

Chishizhi Botuo Fang (Halloysite Hand-pulled Dough Soup Formula) is used to treat cold qi in small intestine and stomach, and dysentery.

赤石脂五两　　碎节如面　　白面七两

Prepare 5 Liang of Chishizhi [赤石脂, Halloysite, Halloysitum Rubrum], grind it into powder. Prepare 7 Liang of flour.

上，以赤石脂末和面，搜作之，煮熟，下葱、酱、五味、腥头，空心食之，三四服皆愈。

Make hand-pulled dough with the above ingredients. Cook it thoroughly and flavor with Chinese green onion, sauce, 5 kinds of seasonings, and condiment. Take on an empty stomach. The disease will be treated after 3 to 4 doses.

食治老人脾胃气冷，肠数痢。黄雌鸡炙方。

Huangciji Zhi Fang (Roast Yellow Hen Formula) is used to treat cold in the spleen and stomach, and dysentery.

黄雌鸡一只，如常法

Prepare one yellow hen and clean it as usual.

上以五椒酱刷炙之令熟，空心渐食之。亦甚补益脏腑。

Flavor with sauce made of seasonings and pepper, and roast it fully. Take it slowly on an empty stomach. It is also very effective to tonify the

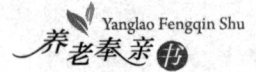

zang-fu organs.

二

食治老人脾胃虚，气频频下痢，瘦乏无力。猪肝煎。

II

Zhugan Jian（Pig Liver Decoction）is used to treat deficiency of qi of the spleen and stomach, frequent dysentery, emaciation, fatigue and lack of strength of the aged.

獖猪肝一具，去膜，切作片，洗去血　好醋一升

Prepare one sliced pig's liver with the membrane removed and 1 Sheng of high-quality vinegar.

上以醋煎肝，微火令泣尽干，即空心常服之。亦明目，温中，除冷气。

Cook the liver gently in vinegar. Take regularly on an empty stomach. It can brighten the eyes, warm the middle internal organs, and eliminates the cold qi.

食治老人脾胃虚弱，冷痛，泻痢无常，不下食。椒面粥方。

Jiaomian Zhou Fang（Pepper Powder Gruel Formula）is used to treat weakness of the spleen and stomach, cold pain, abnormal dysentery, and inability to take food of the aged.

蜀椒一两，熬，捣为末　白面四两

Boil 1 Liang of Sichuan pepper and grind it into powder. Prepare 4

Liang of flour.

上，和椒，拌之令匀，空心食之。日一服，尤佳。

Mix the above ingredients well. Take on an empty stomach. It will be very effective to take once a day.

食治老人冷热不调，下痢赤白，腹痛不止。甘草汤方。

Gancao Tang Fang（Gancao Decoction Formula）is used to treat disorder of cold and heat, red and white dysentery, and abdominal pain of the aged.

甘草一两，切，熬　生姜一两，刮去皮，切　乌豆一合

Slice 1 Liang of Gancao ［甘草, Liquorice Root, Glycyrrhiza uralensis Fisch］ and bring it to a boil. Peel 1 Liang of ginger and prepare 3 He of black beans.

上，以水一升，煎取七合，去滓，空心服之。不过三日服愈。

Boil the above ingredients in 1 Sheng of water until 7 He of liquid remains. Remove the dregs and take on an empty stomach. The patient will be cured in 2 to 3 doses.

食治老人赤白痢，刺痛，不多食，痿瘦。鲫鱼粥方。

Jiyu Zhou Fang（Crucian Carp Gruel Formula）is used to treat red and white dysentery, stabbing pain, poor appetite, and emaciation of the aged.

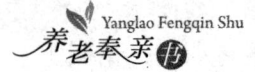

鲫鱼肉七两　青粱米四两　橘皮末一分

It is composed of 7 Liang of crucian carp, 4 Liang of Qingliangmi [青粱米, Seed of Foxtail Millet, Setaria italica], and 1 Fen of orange peel powder.

上相和煮作粥，下五味、椒、酱、葱调和。空心食之，二服。亦治劳，和脏腑。

Make gruel with the above ingredients. Flavor with 5 kinds of seasonings, pepper, sauce, and scallion. Take it twice a day on an empty stomach. It is also effective to treat fatigue and harmonize the zang-fu organs.

食治老人肠胃虚冷，泄痢水谷不分。薤白粥方。

Xiebai Zhou Fang（Longstamen Onion Bulb Gruel Formula）is used to treat deficiency and cold in the intestine and stomach, and diarrhea of the aged.

薤白一握，细切　粳米四合　葱白三合，细切

It is composed of 1 handful of sliced Xiebai [薤白, Longstamen Onion Bulb, Bulbus Allii Macrostemonis], 4 He of polished round-grained rice, and 3 He of sliced scallion.

上相和作羹，下五味、椒、酱、姜，空心食。常作取效。

Make gruel with the above ingredients. Flavor with 5 kinds of seasonings, pepper, sauce, and ginger. Take on an empty stomach. Long-term taking is good for health.

食治老人脾虚气弱，食不消化，泄痢无定。曲末粥方。

Qumo Zhou Fang (Medicated Leaven Powder Gruel Formula) is used to treat spleen deficiency, qi weakness, indigestion, and diarrhea at irregular intervals of the aged.

神曲二两，炙，捣罗为末　青粱米四合，净淘

Prepare 2 Liang of Shenqu [神曲, Medicated Leaven, Massa Medicata Fermentata], roast and grind it into powder. Prepare 4 He of Qingliangmi [青粱米, Seed of Foxtail Millet, Setaria italica] and rinse clean.

上，相和煮粥。空心食之，常三五服，立愈。

Cook gruel with the above ingredients. Take on an empty stomach regularly. Take 3 to 5 doses and it will take effect.

食治老人赤白痢，日夜无度，烦热不止。车前子饮。

Cheqianzi Yin (Cheqianzi Decoction) is used to treat continuous red and white dysentery, and incessant heat with vexation of the aged.

车前子五合，绵裹，用水二升，煎取一升半汁　青粱米三合

It is composed of 5 He of Cheqianzi [车前子, Plantain Seed, Semen Plantaginis] and 3 He of Qingliangmi [青粱米, Seed of Foxtail Millet, Setaria italica］. Wrap Cheqianzi［车前子, Plantain Seed, Semen Plantaginis］with a piece of cotton gauze. Boil in 2 Sheng of water until 1.5 Sheng of liquid remains.

上取煎汁煮作饮。空心食之，日三服。最除热毒。

Decoct the above ingredients. Take it 3 times a day on an empty stomach. It is very effective to expel heat-toxicity.

食治老人痢不止，日渐黄瘦无力，不多食。黍米粥方。

Shumi Zhou Fang（Broomcorn Millet Gruel Formula）is used to treat unstoppable dysentery, yellow complexion, emaciation and flaccidity, and poor appetite of the aged.

黍米四合，净淘　阿胶一两，炙为末

Prepare 4 He of broomcorn millet and wash clean. Roast 1 Liang of Ejiao［阿胶, Ass Hide Glue, Colla Corii Asini］into powder.

上煮粥，临熟下胶末调和。空心食之，一服尤效。

Make gruel with the broomcorn millet, and add the Ejiao powder when it is about to be cooked. Take on an empty stomach. It will be very effective instantly.

食治老人下痢赤白，及水谷不度，腹痛。马齿菜方。

Machicai Fang（Purslane Formula）is used to treat red and white dysentery, stagnation of food and water, and abdominal pain of the aged.

马齿菜一斤，净淘洗

Prepare 1 Jin of Machicai ［马齿菜, Purslane, Portulacae Herba］and wash clean.

上煮令熟，及热，以五味或姜醋渐食之，其功无比。

Cook the above ingredients thoroughly with 5 kinds of seasonings or ginger and vinegar, and take it slowly. It is very effective.

增补方剂
Supplementary Formulas

《太平圣惠方》治血痢，日夜百馀行，宜服此方。

It is recorded in *Taiping Shenghui Fang*（*Taiping Holy Prescriptions for Universal Relief*）this formula.can treat blood dysentery and frequent urination.

葛粉二两　蜜二合

Prepare 2 Liang of Gefen ［葛粉, Pueraria Starch, Puerariae Amylum］and 2 He of honey.

上，以新汲水二中盏，搅令匀，空腹分两度服之。

（卷第九十六·食治一切痢疾诸方）

Fully mix the above ingredients in 2 medium cups (about 10 ml) of fresh water. Take on an empty stomach in 2 times.

(Volume 96·*Formulas to Treat Dysentery*)

苋蒜汤面。食治老人急性赤白痢初起，体质较好，无发热，能食，脉小者。

Amaranth Garlic Noodle with Soup: It is used to treat the aged with good constitution, fair appetite, and small pulse who suffer from acute red and white dysentery at early stage but without fever.

铁苋菜叶鲜者三两，淘净　新鲜大蒜一两，去皮捣汁　白面三两

It is composed of 3 Liang of clean fresh copper-leaf herb, 1 Liang of mashed fresh garlic with the peel removed, and 3 Liang of flour.

上件，先将白面擀成面条，以水两碗，煮沸时下面条待再沸，入铁苋菜叶共煮至熟，下油盐调料做成汤面，加大蒜汁搅和，一次食之。每日二次，以病愈为度。

（经验方）

Roll the dough into noodles. Put the noodles in 2 bowls of water when the water boils. Put the copper-leaf herb in after the second boil. Flavor with oil and salt, and add garlic juice. Take at one time. Take it twice a day until the disease is cured.

(Empirical Formula)

食治烦渴热诸方
Formulas to Treat Vexation, Thirst, and Fever of the Aged with Diet Therapy

一

食治老人烦渴，口干，骨节烦热。枸杞饮方。

I

Gouqi Yin Fang（Wolfberry Decoction Formula）is used to treat vexation and thirst, dryness of the mouth, feverish sensation in the joints of the aged.

枸杞根白皮一升　　小麦一升，净淘　　粳米三合，研

Prepare 1 Sheng of root bark of wolfberry. Rinse 1 Sheng of wheat thoroughly. Grind 3 He of polished round-grained rice into powder.

上以水一斗，煮二味，取七升汁，下米作饮。渴即渐服之。

Boil wolfberry and wheat with 1 Dou of water until 7 Sheng is left. Add polished round-grained rice and take as decoction. It is very effective to take it slowly when thirsty.

食治老人烦渴不止，饮水不定，转渴，舌卷干焦。大麦汤方。

Damai Tang Fang（Barley Decoction Formula）is used to treat persistent polydipsia which is hardly relieved even after drinking water, curled tongue due to dryness.

大麦二升　赤饧二合

It is composed of 2 Sheng of barley and 2 He of brown maltose.

上，以水七升，煎取五升，去滓。下饧调之。渴即服愈。

Boil the barley in 7 Sheng of water until 5 Sheng is left. Remove the dregs before use. Flavor with brown sugar and take the soup when thirsty.

食治老人烦渴，小便黄色无度。黄雌鸡羹方。

Huangciji Geng Fang (Yellow Hen Soup Formula) is used to treat polydipsia, yellow and excessive urine.

黄雌鸡一只，如常法　粳米二合，淘净　葱白一握

Prepare 1 yellow hen and clean it as usual. Rinse 2 He of polished round-grained rice and prepare a handful of Chinese onion stalk.

上，切鸡和煮作羹。下五味，少著盐，空心食之。渐进当效。

Slice the hen and cook with the other ingredients. Flavor with 5 kinds of seasonings and add a little salt. Take on an empty stomach and take it gradually to induce the efficacy.

食治老人消渴热中，饮水不止，小便无度，烦热。猪肚方。

Zhudu Fang (Pork Tripe Formula) is used to treat consumptive thirst, heat strike, incessant drinking of water, frequent urination and heat with vexation of the aged.

猪肚一具，肥者，净洗之　葱白一握　豉五合，绵裹

It is composed of 1 clean fat pork tripe, a handful of scallion, and 5 He of Douchi [豆豉, Fermented Soybean, Semen Sojae Preparatum] wrapped in a piece of cotton gauze.

上，煮烂熟下五味调和，空心，切，渐食之。渴即饮汁。亦治劳热皆差。

Cook the above ingredients thoroughly and flavor with 5 kinds of seasonings. Take it slowly on an empty stomach. Take the soup when thirsty. It is also effective to treat consumptive fever.

二

食治老人烦渴，脏腑干枯，渴不止。野鸡臛方。

II

Yeji Huo Fang (Wild Chicken Broth Formula) is used to treat vexation, thirst, essence exhaustion of the zang-fu organs, and insatiable thirst of the aged.

野鸡一只，如常法　葱白一握　粳米二合，细研

Prepare one wild chicken and clean it as usual. Prepare a handful of Chinese onion stalk and grind 2 He of polished round-grained rice into powder.

上切作相和羹，作臛。下五味、椒、酱，空心食之。常作服佳妙。

Mix the above ingredients to make thick broth. Flavor with 5 kinds of seasonings, pepper, and sauce. Take on an empty stomach. Long-term taking is good for health.

食治老人烦渴，饮水不足，日渐羸瘦困弱。兔头饮方。

Tutou Yin Fang（Rabbit Head Decoction Formula）is used to treat vexation and thirst, not drinking enough water, emaciation, weakness and fatigue of the aged.

兔头一枚，净洗之　豉心五合，绵裹

It is composed of one clean rabbit head and 5 He of Douchi ［豆豉，Fermented Soybean, Semen Sojae Preparatum］ wrapped in a piece of cotton gauze.

上，以水七升，煮取五升汁。渴，即渐饮之，最效。

Boil the above ingredients in 7 Sheng of water until 5 Sheng remains. It would be most effective to take gradually when thirsty.

食治老人消渴烦闷，常热，身体枯燥，黄瘦。牛乳方。

Niuru Fang（Milk Formula）is used to treat consumptive thirst, vexation and oppression, frequent fever, dryness of the skin, yellow complexion and emaciation of the aged.

牛乳一升，真者，微熬

Prepare 1 Sheng of milk and boil on lower flame.

上，空心分为二服。极补益五脏，令人强健光悦。

Take the milk in 2 times on an empty stomach. It is very effective to tonify the five zang-organs, keep fit and refine the complexion.

食治老人消渴、壮热、燥不安，兼无力。青粱米饮方。

Qingliangmi Yin Fang（Qingliangmi Decoction Formula）is used to treat consumptive thirst, high fever, vexation, and flaccidity of the aged.

青粱米一升，净洗淘之，研令细

Wash 1 Sheng of Qingliangmi ［青粱米 , Seed of Foxtail Millet, Setaria italica］, and grind into powder finely.

上，以水三升，和煮之。渴，即渐服之。极治热，燥并除。

Boil the above ingredients in 3 Sheng of water. Take gradually when thirsty. It is very effective to clear heat and dryness.

食治老人消渴热中，饮水无度，常若不足。青豆方。

Qingdou Fang（Green Soya Bean Decoction Formula）is used to treat consumptive thirst, heat stroke and excessive drinking of water but still thirsty of the aged.

青豆二斤，净淘

It is composed of 2 Jin of green soya beans rinsed clean.

上，煮令烂熟。空心，饥即食之。渴即饮汁。或作粥食之，任性益佳。

Cook the above ingredients thoroughly. Take on an empty stomach or take when hungry. Take the soup when thirsty. Or take as gruel as much as you like.

食治老人消渴，烦热，心神狂乱，躁闷不安。冬瓜羹方。

Donggua Geng Fang（White Gourd Soup Formula）is used to treat consumptive thirst, heat with vexation, mania, and restlessness of the aged.

冬瓜半斤，去皮　豉心二合，绵裹　葱白半握

It is composed of 0.5 Jin of peeled white gourd, 2 He of Douchi［豆豉, Fermented Soybean, Semen Sojae Preparatum］wrapped in a piece of cotton gauze, and half a handful of scallion.

上，以和煮作羹。下五味调和，空心食之。常作粥佳。

Cook gruel with the above ingredients. Flavor with 5 kinds of seasonings and take on an empty stomach. It is appropriate to be taken as gruel often.

食治老人消渴消中，饮水不足，五脏干枯。芦根饮子。

Hugen Yinzi（Reed Rhizome Decoction）is used to treat consumptive thirst, center dispersion, insufficiency of drinking water, essence exhaustion of the five zang-organs of the aged.

芦根切，一升，水一斗，煎取七升半　青粱米五合

Sclice 1 Sheng of Lugen〔芦根, phragmites, Phragmitis Rhizoma〕. Boil it in 1 Dou of water until 7.5 Sheng of liquid remains. Prepare 5 He of Qingliangmi〔青粱米, Seed of Foxtail Millet, Setaria italica〕.

上，以煎煮饮，空心食之。渐进为度，益效。忌咸食、炙肉、熟面等。

Boil the above ingredients and take on an empty stomach. It is effective to take it slowly. It is contraindicated with Xianshi（a kind of food like roll made of wheat and vegetables popular in Northern China）, roast meat and cooked flour product.

食治老人消渴，诸药不差，黄瘦力弱。鹿头方。

Lutou Fang（Deer Head Formula）is used to treat consumptive thirst, yellow complexion, emaciation and flaccidity of the aged.

鹿头一枚，炮去毛，净洗之

Prepare one deer head, remove its hair with fire and wash clean.

上，煮令烂熟。空心，日以五味食之，并服汁极效。

Cook the above ingredients thoroughly. Flavor with 5 kinds of seasonings and take on an empty stomach daily. It would be effective to take the soup at the same time.

增补方剂
Supplementary Formulas

《太平圣惠方》治消渴。瓜蒌粉方。

It is recorded in *Taiping Shenghui Fang*（*Taiping Holy Prescriptions for Universal Relief*）that Trichosanthes powder formula can be used to treat consumptive thirst.

瓜蒌根多取，削去皮。二月、三月、八月、九月造佳

Take a lot of Gualougen ［瓜蒌根，Trichosanthes Root, Trichosanthis Radix］ and peel. Those grown in February, March, August and September are of the best quality.

上，于新瓦中磨讫，以水淘，生绢袋摆，如造米粉法，曝干。热渴时，冷水调下一钱服之，大效。

（卷十六·食治三痟诸方）

Grind the above ingredients on new tile and wash clean. Put it in a kiginu bag and process it like making rice noodles. Dry it in the sun. Dissolve 1 Qian of the powder in cold water and take it when thirsty. It is very effective.

（Volume 16 · *Formulas to Treat Three Consumptive Thirsts with Diet Therapy*）

《太平圣惠方》治心脏烦热，止渴除口干，散积血，极效方。

It is recorded in *Taiping Shenghui Fang*（*Taiping Holy Prescriptions for Universal Relief*）that this formula is effective to treat feverish sensation in the heart, relieve thirst and dryness of the mouth, and remove blood stasis.

藕半斤，去皮，绞取汁。

Prepare half Jin of lotus root, peel and extract juice.

上以蜜一合相和，服之。

（卷十六·食治烦热诸方）

Mix the above ingredients with 1 He of honey and take it.

（Volume 16 · *Formulas to Treat Vexing Fever with Diet Therapy*）

食治水气诸方
Formulas to Treat Edema Disease of the Aged with Diet Therapy

一

食治老人水气病，身体肿，闷满气急，不能食，皮肤欲裂，四肢常疼，不可屈伸。鲤鱼臛方。

I

Liyu Huo Fang（Carp Broth Formula）is used to treat edema disease, swelling, oppression and fullness, rapid breathing, absence of food intake, cracking of the skin, pain in the limbs, inhibited bending and stretching of the aged.

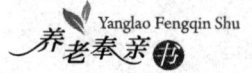

鲤鱼肉十两　葱白一握　麻子一升，熬，细研

Prepare 10 Liang of carp meat and a handful of Chinese onion stalk. Boil 1 Sheng of cannabis fruit and grind thoroughly.

上以水滤麻子汁，和煮作臛，下五味、椒、姜调和，空心时渐食之。常服尤佳。

Sieve cannabis fruit juice with water, and mix it with the above ingredients to make sauce. Flavor with 5 kinds of seasonings, pepper, and ginger. Take on an empty stomach. Long-term taking is good for health.

食治老人水气病，四肢肿闷沉重，喘息不安。水牛肉方。

Shuiniurou Fang（Buffalo Formula）is used to treat edema disease, heaviness and swelling in the limbs, and restless panting of the aged.

水牛肉一斤，鲜

Prepare 1 Jin of fresh buffalo meat.

上，蒸令烂熟。空心，切，以五味、姜、醋。渐食之，任性为佳。

Steam the meat until it's well cooked. Slice the meat and flavor with ginger, vinegar and 5 kinds of seasonings. Take on an empty stomach slowly and take as much as you like.

食治老人水气浮肿，身、皮肤燥痒，气急，不能下食，心腹胀满，气欲绝。貒肉羹方。

Tuanrougeng Fang (Wild Boar Meat Soup Formula) is used to treat edema, itchy skin, rapid breathing, inability to take food, distention and fullness in the heart and abdomen.

貒肉一斤，细切　葱白半握，切　粳米三合，淅

It is composed of 1 Jin of sliced wild boar meat, half a handful of sliced Chinese onion stalk, and 3 He of polished round-grained rice.

上，和煮作羹。下五味、椒、姜，空心常食之，最验。

Cook gruel with the above ingredients. Flavor with 5 kinds of seasonings, pepper, and ginger. It is effective to take it regularly on an empty stomach.

食治老人水气肿满，身体疼痛，不能食。麻子粥方。

Mazizhou Fang (Cannabis Fruit Gruel Formula) is used to treat edema, swelling and fullness, pain in the body, and inability to take food of the aged.

冬麻子一升，研取汁　鲤鱼肉七两，切

Boil 1 Sheng of Dongmazi [冬麻子, Cannabis Fruit, Cannabis Fructus], grind and then filter to get the juice. Slice 7 Liang of carp.

上，取麻子汁，下米四合，和鱼煮作粥。以五味、葱、椒，空心食，日一服。频作皆愈。

Make gruel with the above ingredients and 4 He of rice. Flavor with 5 kinds of seasonings, green Chinese onion and pepper. Take on an empty stomach once a day. Long-term taking can cure the disease.

食治老人水气胀闷，手足浮肿，气急烦满。赤豆方。

Chidou Fang（Red Bean Formula）is used to treat edema, distention and oppression, dropsy of hands and feet, rapid breathing, vexation and fullness of the aged.

赤小豆三升，淘净　樟柳根好者，切，一升

Prepare and wash 3 Sheng of red bean. Slice 1 Jin of camphor willow root of good quality.

上和豆煮烂熟。空心常食豆。渴即饮汁。勿别杂食，服三二服立效。

Cook the above ingredients thoroughly. Take it on an empty stomach. Take the soup when thirsty. Do not take anything else. It will be effective after taking 2 to 3 doses.

食治老人水气，面肿腹胀，喘乏不安，转动不得，手足不仁，身体重困或疼痛。郁李仁粥方。

Yuliren Zhou Fang（Bush Cherry Kernel Gruel Formula）is used to treat edema, swollen face, abdominal distention, panting and fatigue, inability to turn sides, numbness of the limbs, and heaviness and pain in the body of the aged.

郁李仁二两，研，以水滤取汁　薏苡仁五合，淘

Prepare 2 Liang of Yuliren［郁李仁, Bush Cherry Kernel, Pruni Semen］, grind and then filter to get the juice. Prepare 5 He of Yiyiren［薏苡仁, Coix Seed, Semen Coicis］and wash clean.

上以煎汁作粥。空心食之，日二服。常立效。

Make gruel with the above ingredients. Take on an empty stomach twice a day. Regular taking will be very effective.

食治老人水气，面目、手足浮肿，腹胀，风急。桑白皮饮。

Sangbaipi Yin（White Mulberry Root-bark Decoction）is used to treat edema, dropsy of the face and limbs, abdominal distention, and acute wind syndrome of the aged.

桑白皮切四两，切　青粱米四合，研

Slice 4 Liang of Sangbaipi［桑白皮, White Mulberry Root-bark, Cortex Mori］. Prepare 4 He of Qingliangmi［青粱米, Seed of Foxtail Millet, Setaria italica］and grind it into powder.

上，以桑汁煮作饮，空心渐食，常服尤佳益。

Boil the above ingredients with the juice of white mulberry root-bark. Take it slowly on an empty stomach. Long-term taking is good for health.

食治老人水气疾，心腹胀满，四肢烦疼、无力。白煮鲤鱼方。

Baizhu Liyu Fang (Boiled Carp formula) is used to treat edema, distention and fullness in the heart region and abdomen, vexing pain in the limbs and flaccidity of the aged.

鲤鱼一头重二斤，如常法　橘皮二两

Prepare 2 Jin of carp and process as usual. Prepare 2 Liang of tangerine peel.

上，和煮令烂熟。空心，以二味少著盐食之。常服并饮少许汁，将理为验。

Cook the above ingredients thoroughly. Flavor with a pinch of salt, and take on an empty stomach. Take regularly and drink a little soup. A good rest and regulation will make it effective.

食治水气肿满，手足俱肿，心烦，满闷，无力。大豆方。

Dadou Fang (Soy Bean Formula) is used to treat edema, swelling and fullness, swollen limbs, heart vexation, fullness and oppression and lack of strength of the aged.

大豆二升　白术二两　鲤鱼肉一斤

It is composed of 2 Sheng of soy beans, 2 Liang of Baizhu [白术, Argehead Atractylodes Rhizome, Rhizoma Atractylodis Macrocephalae], and 1 Jin of carp.

上，以水和煮，令豆烂熟，空心常食之鱼豆，饮其汁，尤佳。

Boil the above ingredients in water. Cook the beans thoroughly. Take on an empty stomach regularly. It is very beneficial to drink the soup.

食治老人水气，身体虚肿，面目虚胀。水牛皮方。

Shuiniupi Fang（Buffalo Hide Formula）is used to treat edema disease, swelling limbs and face of the aged.

水牛皮二斤，刮去毛，净洗　橘皮一两

Prepare 2 Jin of buffalo hide, shave the hair and wash it clean. Prepare 1 Liang of tangerine peel.

上，相和，煮令烂熟。切，以生姜、醋、五味渐食之。常作尤益。

Cook all the above ingredients thoroughly. Slice and flavor with fresh ginger, vinegar, and 5 kinds of seasonings. Long-term taking of it is good for health.

食治喘嗽诸方
Formulas to Treat Panting and Cough of the Aged with Diet Therapy

一

食治老人上，气急，喘息不得，坐卧不安。猪颐酒方。

Zhuyi Jiu Fang (Pig's Cheek Wine Formula) is used to treat tachypnea, inability to breathe, restlessness of the aged.

猪颐三具，细切　　青州枣三十枚

Prepare 3 sliced pig's cheek and 30 Chinese dates from Qingzhou.

上，以酒三升浸之。若秋冬三五日，春夏一二日，密封头，以布绞去滓。空心，温，任性渐服之。极验。忌咸热。

Soak the above ingredients in 3 Sheng of wine for 3 to 5 days in autumn or winter, or one to 2 days in spring or summer. Seal tight and remove the dregs with a piece of cloth. Warm it and take on an empty stomach. Take as much as you like slowly. It is very effective. It is contraindicated with salty and hot food.

食治老人上气咳嗽，胸中妨满，急喘。桃仁粥方。

Taoren Zhou Fang (Peach Seed Gruel Formula) is used to treat cough due to qi ascent, fullness and oppression in the chest, and rapid panting of the aged.

桃仁三两，去皮尖，研　　青粱米二合，净淘

Prepare 3 Liang of Taoren ［桃仁, peach seed, Semen Persicae］, remove the peel and pointed part, then grind into powder. Wash 2 He of Qingliangmi ［青粱米, Seed of Foxtail Millet, Setaria italica］.

上调桃仁和米煮作粥。空心食之，日一服尤益。

Cook the above ingredients to make gruel. It is very effective to take on an empty stomach once a day.

食治老人上气咳嗽，烦热，干燥，不能食。饧煎方。

Xingjian Fang（Maltose Decoction Formula）is used to treat cough due to qi ascent, heat with vexation, dryness, inability to take food of the aged.

寒食饧四两　干地黄生者，汁一升　白蜜三合

It is composed of 4 Liang of maltose made on Cold Food Festival, 1 Sheng of Shengdihuang［生地黄，Unprocessed Rehmannia Root, Radix Rehmanniae Recens］juice. Prepare 3 He of white honey.

上相和，微火煎之，令稠。即空心，每日含半匙，细咽汁。食后亦服。除热最效。

Mix the above ingredients and decoct with low fire until it is thick. Take on an empty stomach. Keep half a spoon of it in mouth once a day and swallow slowly. It can also be taken after meal. It is very effective to eliminate heat.

食治老人上喘、咳嗽，身体壮热，口干渴燥。猪脂方。

Zhuzhi Fang（Pig Fat Formula）is used to treat reverse panting, cough, vigorous heat, dryness and thirst of the mouth of the aged.

猪肪脂一斤，切，作脔

Prepare 1 Jin of pig's fat and slice.

上于沸汤中投煮之。空心，以五味渐食之。其效不可比，补劳，治百病。

Add the above ingredients into boiled soup. Take on an empty stomach. Flavor it with 5 kinds of seasonings and take it slowly. It is effective to treat consumptive disease and many other kinds of diseases.

食治老人上喘咳嗽，气急，面目浮肿，坐卧不得。苏煎方。

Sujian Fang（Perilla Decoction Formula）is used to treat reverse panting, cough, rapid breathing, swelling in the face, and restlessness of the aged.

土苏四两　鹿髓三合　生地黄汁一升

It is composed of 4 Liang of Tusu［土苏, Perilla Leaf, Folium Perillae］, 3 He of deer's marrow, and 1 Sheng of Shengdihuang［生地黄, Unprocessed Rehmannia Root, Radix Rehmanniae Recens］juice.

上相和，微火煎之如饧即止。空心及食后，常含半匙，细咽汁。三两日即差。

Mix the above ingredients up and decoct with low heat until thick like maltose. Take on an empty stomach or after meal. Keep half a spoon of it in the mouth and swallow slowly. The disease can be cured in 2 or 3 days.

食治老人气急胸膈逆满，食饮不下。枣煎方。

Zaojian Fang (Chinese Date Decoction Formula) is used to treat qi ascent, rapid breathing chest and diaphragm counter-flow fullness, inability to get down.

青州枣三十枚，大者，去核　土苏三两　饧二合

Prepare 30 big Chinese dates from Qingzhou and remove the pit. Prepare 3 Liang of Tusu [土苏, Perilla Leaf, Folium Perillae] and 2 He of maltose.

上相和，微火温令消，即下枣搅之，相和，以微火煎，令苏饧泣尽即止。每食止即啖一二枚，渐渐咽汁为佳。忌咸、热、炙肉。

Mix the above ingredients up and cook gently until the maltose melts. Put Chinese dates in and stir well. Fry until all Tusu [土苏, Perilla Leaf, Folium Perillae] and maltose melts. Take 1 or 2 Chinese dates after each meal. It is good to swallow the juice slowly. It is contraindicated with salty food, hot food, and roasted meat.

食治老人咳嗽，胸胁引痛，即多见唾涕。燠梨方。

Yuli Fang (Hot Pear Formula) is used to treat cough that induces pain in rib-sides, drool and spittle of the aged.

黄梨一大颗，刺作五十孔　蜀椒五十粒　面二两

Prick 50 holes in a big yellow pear and put one Sichuan pepper in each hole. Prepare 2 Liang of flour.

上，以蜀椒每孔内一颗，软面软裹，放于塘灰火中，候煨令熟。去面，冷，空心切食，用二三服尤佳。不当，及热食之益甚，须羊肚肝羹治之。

Wrap the pear in batter and put it in embers until cooked. Remove the batter and cool. Slice it and take on an empty stomach. It is effective to take 2 to 3 times. If the disease is worsened when taking hot food, it can be treated with Lamb Tripe and Liver Soup.

食治老人上气咳嗽，喘急，烦热，不下食，食即吐逆，腹胀满。姜糖煎方。

Jiangtang Jian Fang（Ginger Sugar Decoction Formula）is used to treat cough due to qi ascent, rapid breathing, heat with vexation, inability to take food, vomiting and qi counter-flow after eating, abdominal distention and fullness of the aged.

生姜汁五两　砂糖四两

It is composed of 5 Liang of fresh ginger juice and 4 Liang of granulated sugar.

上相和，微火温之。一二十沸即止。每度含半匙，渐渐下汁。

Put all the above ingredients together and steam it with low fire. It will be well done after 10 to 20 times of boiling. Take half a spoon of it once slowly.

食治老人咳嗽，虚弱，口舌干燥，涕唾浓粘。甘蔗粥方。

Ganzhe Zhou Fang（Sugarcane Gruel Formula）is used to treat cough, deficiency, dryness of the mouth and tongue, thick saliva and nasal mucus of the aged.

甘蔗汁一升半　青粱米四合，净淘

Prepare 1.5 Sheng of Sugarcane juice. Wash 4 He of Qingliangmi［青粱米, Seed of Foxtail Millet, Setaria italica］.

上，以蔗汁煮粥，空心渐食之，日一二服。极润心肺。

Make gruel with the above ingredients. Take on an empty stomach gradually. Take it once or twice a day. It is effective to moisten the lung and heart.

食治老人上气、热，咳嗽引心腹痛，满闷。桃仁煎方。

Taoren Jian Fang（Peach Seed Decoction Formula）is used to treat qi ascent, heat, pain in heart region and abdomen due to cough, fullness and oppression of the aged.

桃仁二两，去皮尖，熬末　赤饧四合

Prepare 2 Liang of Taoren ［桃仁, peach seed, Semen Persicae］, peel and remove the pointed part. Bring it to a boil and grind into powder. Prepare 4 He of brown maltose.

上相和，微煎三五沸即止。空心，每度含少许，渐渐咽汁尤益。

Mix the above ingredients, decoct until boiling for 3 to 5 times. Take it on an empty stomach, keep a little in the mouth and swallow slowly.

食治老人咳嗽、烦热，或唾血、气急，不能食。地黄饮方。

Dihuang Yin Fang（Rehmannia Decoction Formula）is used to treat cough, heat with vexation, spitting of blood, rapid breathing and inability to take food.

生地黄半斤，研如水取汁

Prepare half Jin of Shengdihuang ［生地黄, Unprocessed Rehmannia Root, Radix Rehmanniae Recens］, grind and get the juice.

上，以地黄汁煎作膏，空心渐食之，日一服。极效。

Decoct the juice to paste. Take on an empty stomach gradually once a day. It is very effective.

增补方剂
Supplementary Formulas

《太平圣惠方》治肺气,疗虚羸,喘息促急,咳嗽等。杏仁粥方。

According to *Taiping Shenghui Fang*（*Taiping Holy Prescriptions for Universal Relief*）, apricot seed gruel formula can be used to treat diseases involving the lung, deficiency and emaciation, rapid panting, coughing, etc.

杏仁二十一枚,汤浸去皮尖双仁,研,以三合黄牛乳投绞取汁　枣七枚,去核　粳米二合　桑白皮一两,锉　生姜一分,切

Prepare twenty-one Xingren ［杏仁, Bitter Apricot Seed, Semen Armeniacae Amarum］. Soak in water and peel. Remove the pointed parts and grind. Mix the powder with 3 He of milk of yellow cattle. Prepare 7 Chinese dates and remove the pit. Prepare 2 He of polished round-grained rice, 1 Liang of filed Sangbaipi ［桑白皮, White Mulberry Root-bark, Cortex Mori］, and 1 Fen of sliced fresh ginger.

上,以水三大盏,先煮桑根白皮、姜、枣等,取汁三盏。将米煮粥,候临熟,入杏仁汁,更煮五七沸。粥成,不计时候食之。

Boil the above ingredients in 3 cups of water. Boil Sanggen Baipi ［桑根白皮, mulberry bark, Mori Cortex］, ginger, and Chinese dates first to get 3 cups of decoction. Cook rice gruel and put Xingren ［杏仁, Bitter Apricot Seed, Semen Armeniacae Amarum］ juice in when it is about to be cooked. Decoct until boiling for 3 to 5 times. Take it anytime.

食治老人阳虚感寒，咳嗽喘息不能卧，咯吐清白稀痰，微热少汗，肢冷，脉沉细者。猪肺汤方。

Pig lung soup formula is used to treat cold due to yang deficiency, inability to lie due to coughing and panting, vomiting of white and clear phlegm, slight fever, absence of sweating, and cold limbs of the aged with sunken and thin pulse.

猪肺新鲜者，一具，洗净　麻黄五钱　细辛五钱　附子五钱，炮，去皮脐

Prepare a fresh pig lung and wash clean. Prepare 5 Qian of Mahuang［麻黄, Ephedra, Herba Ephedrae］, 5 Qian of Xixin ［细辛, Asarum, Asarum sieboldii Miq.］, and 5 Qian of processed Fuzi ［附子, Aconite, Radix Aconiti Praeparata］ with the peel and navel removed.

上以水六碗，先煎麻黄、细辛、附子至五碗，去药渣及上沫。再将猪肺切块入药液中共煮至熟，加盐酱五味椒姜，分六次食之，每日早晚各一次。

Decoct the above ingredients in 6 bowls of water, decoct Mahuang ［麻黄, Ephedra, Herba Ephedrae］, Xixin ［细辛, Asarum, Asarum sieboldii Miq.］, and Fuzi ［附子, Aconite, Radix Aconiti Praeparata］ until 5 bowls of water remains, remove the dregs and skim off scum. Chop the pig lung and put them in the decoction to cook together. Flavor with salt, 5 kinds of seasonings, pepper, and ginger. Take in 6 separated doses. Take one dose in the morning and one in the evening.

食治老人久病喘息，咳嗽，吐少量清稀痰，动则喘甚，张口抬肩，心悸少寐，虚羸消瘦，舌淡，两寸尺脉弱。炖胎盘方。

Placenta formula is used to treat enduring panting, cough, clear and thin phlegm, panting on exertion, gaping mouth and raised shoulders, palpitation, reduced sleep, emaciation due to deficiency of the aged with pale tongue coating and weakness of Cun and Chi pulse.

胎盘一具，取新鲜者，清水漂净污血，切块　杏仁五钱，去皮尖　百合一两，渍一宿，当白沫出，去其水　胡桃仁净者，一两。

Prepare and wash 1 fresh placenta and cut it up. Prepare 5 Qian of Xingren ［杏仁，Bitter Apricot Seed, Semen Armeniacae Amarum］, peel and remove the pointed parts. Soak 1 Liang of Baihe ［百合，lily bulb, Lilium brownii var. viridulum Baker］ for one night and drain the foam. Prepare 1 Liang of Hutaoren ［胡桃仁，walnut, Juglandis Semen］ washed clean.

上四味，加水四碗，熟炖至两碗，入盐酱等调味品，分两次食之，早晚各服一次。

（经验方）

Stew the above ingredients in 4 bowls of water until 2 bowls are left. Flavor with salt and other seasonings. Take it in 2 doses in the morning and evening.

（Empirical Formula）

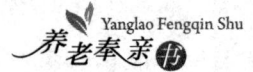

食治老人咳嗽，咯吐黄脓痰，口苦舌干，大便干燥，微热，或鼻塞流浊涕，舌质红，脉沉数。猪胆蜂浆方。

Pig gallbladder and honey formula is used to treat cough, yellow phlegm with pus, bitter taste in the mouth and dry tongue, dryness of the stool, slight fever, stuffy nose, thick yellow snivel of the aged with red tongue coating, deep and rapid pulse.

猪胆一枚，新鲜者，取胆汁　　生蜂蜜二斤

Prepare 1 fresh pig gallbladder and get the bile. Prepare 2 Jin of raw honey.

上二味混合，加热至熟。每日早晚空心时，以开水送服二匙。

（经验方）

Mix up the above ingredients and boil thoroughly. Take on an empty stomach in the morning and evening every day. Take 2 spoons with lukewarm water each time.

（Empirical Formula）

食治脚气诸方
Formulas to Treat Beriberi of the Aged with Diet Therapy

一

食治老人脚气，烦热，流肿入膝，满闷。猪肚生方。

I

Zhudu Sheng Fang (Fresh Pork Tripe Formula) is used to treat beriberi, heat with vexation, purulent kneel discharge, fullness and oppression of the aged.

猪肚一具，肥者细切作生

Prepare one fresh fat pork tripe and slice thinly.

上，以水洗，布绞令干。好蒜、醋、椒、酱、五味，空心常食之。亦治热劳，补益效。

Wash the above ingredients clean and dry with a piece of cloth. Flavor with garlic, vinegar, pepper, sauce and 5 kinds of seasonings. Take on an empty stomach regularly. It can also be used to treat consumptive disease due to heat and it has good tonifying function.

食治老人脚气毒闷，身体不任，行履不能。紫苏粥方。

Zisu Zhou Fang (Perilla Gruel Formula) is used to treat beriberi with toxic and vexed symptoms, insensitivity of the body, inability to walk of the aged.

紫苏子五合，熬，研细，以水投取汁　粳米四合，净淘

Boil 5 He of Zisuzi [紫苏子, Perilla Fruit, Perillae Fructus] and grind it thoroughly. Put it into water to get the juice. Wash 4 He of polished round-grained rice.

上煮作粥，临熟下苏汁调之。空心而食之，日一服。亦温中。

Make gruel with the above ingredients. Add perilla juice when it is nearly cooked. Take on an empty stomach once a day. It is also effective to warm the middle internal organs.

食治老人脚气，逆闷，呕吐，冲心，不能下食。猪肾生方。

Zhushen Sheng Fang (Fresh Pig-Kidney Formula) is used to treat beriberi, counter-flow of qi, chest distress, vomiting, stagnation of the heart, and inability to take food of the aged.

猪肾二只，去膜细切，作生

Prepare 2 pig kidneys, remove the membrane and slice thinly.

上，以蒜、醋、五味空心食之，日一服佳极。

Flavor with garlic, vinegar and 5 kinds of seasonings. Take on an empty stomach. It is effective to take it once a day.

食治老人脚气冲逆，身肿脚肿，大小便秘涩不通，气息喘急，食饮不下。郁李仁饮方。

Yuliren Yin Fang (Bush Cherry Kernel drink Formula) is used to treat beriberi with symptom of reverse flow of qi, swelling of the body and feet, inhibited urination, constipation, panting and inability to take food of the aged.

郁李仁二两，细研，以水滤取汁　　薏苡仁四合，淘研，破

Prepare 2 Liang of Yuliren［郁李仁, Bush Cherry Kernel, Pruni Semen］, grind thoroughly with the juice preserved. Prepare 4 He of Yiyiren［薏苡仁, Coix Seed, Semen Coicis］, wash and grind into powder.

上，以相和煮饮，空心食之。一二服极验。

Decoct the above ingredients and take on an empty stomach. It will be effective after 1 to 2 doses.

食治老人脚气逆，心闷烦躁，心神狂误。鲤鱼臛方。

Liyu Huo Fang（Carp Broth Formula）is used to treat beriberi with symptom of reverse flow of qi, vexation and agitation, restlessness of the aged.

鲤鱼一斤，取肉　　蓴菜四两　　粳米三合，研

It is composed of 1 Jin of carp, 4 Liang of Pocai［蓴菜, Water Shield, Brasenia schreberi J. F. Gmel.］, and 3 He of polished round-grained rice grounded into powder.

上切，以葱白一握，相和煮臛。下五味、椒、姜调和，空心食之。常服亦治水气。

Boil the above ingredients into broth, add a handful of scallion. Flavor with 5 kinds of seasonings, pepper, and ginger. Take on an empty stomach.

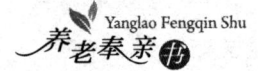

Regular taking can also treat edema.

食治老人脚气，烦闷或吐逆，不下食，痹弱。麻子粥方。

Mazi Zhou Fang（Cannabis Fruit Gruel Formula）is used to treat beriberi, vexation and oppression or vomiting and counterflow, inability to take food, and weakness and paralysis of the aged.

麻子一斤，熬研，水滤取汁　　粳米四合，净淘

Boil 1 Jin of Mazi［麻子, Cannabis Fruit, Cannabis Fructus］and then grind with the juice preserved. Prepare 4 He of polished round-grained rice and wash clean.

上，以麻子汁作粥。空心食之，日一服，尤益。亦中治冷气。

Make gruel with the above ingredients and take on an empty stomach once a day. It also can be used to treat cold syndrome.

食治老人脚气烦燥，或逆，心间愦，呕逆。水牛头方。

Shuiniutou Fang（Buffalo Head Formula）is used to treat beriberi, vexation and agitation in the heart, and vomiting of the aged.

水牛头一枚，炮去毛，洗之

Prepare 1 buffalo head, remove its hair with fire and wash clean.

上煮令烂熟，切。以姜、醋、五味，空心渐渐食之，皆效。

Boil it thoroughly and slice it. Flavor with ginger, vinegar, and 5 kinds of seasonings, Take it slowly on an empty stomach.

食治老人脚气毒冲心，身面浮肿、气急。熊肉腌方。

Xiongrou Yan Fang（Salted Bear Meat Formula）is used to treat beriberi, toxin surging up into the heart, puffy swelling in the face and body, and rapid breathing of the aged.

熊肉二斤，肥者，切作块

Cut 2 Jin of fat bear meat into pieces.

上切。以五味作腌腊，空心，日炙食之。亦可作羹粥，任性食之，极效。

Slice the above ingredients. Flavor with 5 kinds of seasonings and dry it in the sun. Roast and take on an empty stomach. It can also be taken as gruel. Take as much as one likes and it is effective.

食治老人脚气攻心，烦闷，胸腹胀满。乌鸡羹方。

Wuji Geng Fang（Black Chicken Soup Formula）is used to treat beriberi attacking the heart, vexation and fullness, and distention in the chest and abdomen of the aged.

乌鸡一只，治如常法　葱白一握，细切　米二合，研

Prepare 1 black chicken and clean it as usual. Prepare a handful of Chinese onion stalk and slice thinly, grand 2 He of ground rice.

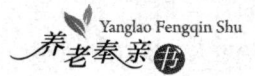

上，煮令熟。空心，切。以五味作羹，常食之为佳。

Boil all the above ingredients. Take on an empty stomach. Make soup with 5 kinds of seasonings. Long-term taking is good for health.

食治老人脚气，肾虚气损，脚膝无力，困乏。生栗方。

Shengli Fang（Fresh Chestnut Formula）is used to treat beriberi, kidney vacuity, qi deficiency, lassitude in feet and knees, and fatigue of the aged.

生栗一斤，以蒸熟，透风处悬令干

Steam 1 Jin of fresh chestnuts and then hang them in a ventilated place to dry.

上，以每日空心常食十颗。极治脚气，不测有功。

Take 10 chestnuts on an empty stomach every day. It is very effective to treat beriberi.

食治老人脚气烦痹，缓弱不随，行履不能。猪肾粥方。

Zhushen Zhou Fang（Pig kidney Gruel Formula）is used to treat foot lichen, vexation and oppression impediment, hemiplegia and inability to walk.

猪肾二双，去膜，切细　粳米四合，淘　葱白半握

Prepare 4 pig kidneys, remove the membrane and slice thinly. Wash

4 He of polished round-grained rice and prepare half a handful of Chinese onion stalk.

上，和煮作粥。下五味、椒、姜，空心食之。日一服，最验。

Cook gruel with the above ingredients. Flavor with 5 kinds of seasonings, pepper, and ginger. Take on an empty stomach. It is very effective to take once a day.

食治老人脚气痹弱，五缓六急，烦躁不安。豉心酒方。

Chixin Jiu Fang (Fermented Soy Bean Wine Formula) is used to treat beriberi, weakness and paralysis, wind-cold obstruction, and vexation and agitation of the aged.

豉心一升，九蒸九晒为佳　　酒五升

Prepare 1 Sheng of fermented soybeans cores which has been steamed and dried for many times. Prepare 5 Sheng of wine.

上，以酒浸一二日。空心，任意温服三盏，极效。

Soak the fermented soybeans cores in wine for 1 to 2 days. Take on an empty stomach. It is very effective to take 3 small cups of it at will while it's hot.

增补方剂

Supplementary Formulas

《太平圣惠方》治脚气，心腹烦闷。槟榔粥方。

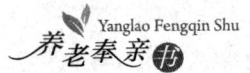

It is recorded in *Taiping Shenghui Fang*（*Taiping Holy Prescriptions for Universal Relief*）that Areca-nut gruel formula can be used to treat beriberi, vexation and oppression in the heart and abdomen.

槟榔一枚，熟水磨令尽　　生姜汁半两　　蜜半合　　粳米二合

Prepare 1 Binglang ［槟榔, Areca Seed, Semen Arecae］, and grind it with boiled water. Prepare half Liang of fresh ginger juice, half He of honey, and 2 He of polished round-grained rice.

上，以水一大盏半，先将米煮粥，欲熟，次下槟榔汁等，更煮令熟，空腹顿服。

（卷第九十七）

Boil the above ingredients in 1.5 cups of water. Make gruel with the rice first, then add areca nut juice when it is about to be cooked. Bring it to another boil. Take on an empty stomach at a draught.

（Volume 97）

食治诸淋方

Formulas to Treat Stranguria of the Aged with Diet Therapy

食治老人五淋，小便涩痛，常频不利，烦热。麻子粥方。

Mazi Zhou Fang（Linseed Gruel Formula）is used to treat 5 types of stranguria with inhibited painful urination, frequent urine, inhibited urination and heat with vexation of the aged.

麻子五合，熬研，水滤取汁　　青粱米四合，淘之

Boil and grind 5 He of linseed. Sieve the juice. Wash 4 He of Qingliangmi［青粱米, Seed of Foxtail Millet, Setaria italica］.

上，以麻子汁煮作粥，空心渐食之，一日二服，常益佳。

Make gruel with the above ingredients. Take it slowly on an empty stomach twice a day.

食治老人淋病，小便不通利，秘涩少痛。榆皮索饼方。

Yupi Suobing Fang（Dwarf Elm Bark Noodle Formula）is used to treat stranguria, inhibited urination, and astringent urination of the aged.

榆皮二两，切，用水三升，煮取一升半汁　　白面六两

Slice 2 Liang of dwarf elm bark, then boil in 3 Sheng of water one and a half Sheng of decoction remains. Prepare 6 Liang of flour.

上，搜面作之，于榆汁拌煮。下五味、葱、椒，空心食之。常三五服，极利水道。

Make noodle with the flour and cook it with the decoction of dwarf elm bark. Flavor with 5 kinds of seasonings, Chinese onion, and pepper. Take on an empty stomach. Taking 3 or 5 doses will take effect and free the water passages inside the body.

食治老人五淋病，身体烦热，小便痛、不利。浆水饮。

Jiangshui Yin（Millet Water Decoction）is used to treat 5 types of stranguria, feverish sensation of the body, painful and inhibited urination.

浆水三升，酸美者　青粱米三合，研

Prepare 3 Sheng of millet sour water. Grind 3 He of Qingliangmi ［青粱米, Seed of Foxtail Millet, Setaria italica］.

上，煮作饮。空心，渐饮之，日二三服。亦宣利效。

Boil the above ingredients into decoction. Take on an empty stomach gradually. Take 2 or 3 doses one day. It is also effective to diffuse and disinhibit.

食治老人淋，小便秘涩，烦热燥痛，四肢寒栗。葵菜羹方。

Kuicai Geng Fang（Mallow Soup Formula）is used to treat stranguria, rough urination, heat with vexation, pain due to dryness, and cold limbs of the aged.

葵菜四两，切　青粱米三合，研　葱白一握

Prepare 4 Liang of mallow. Prepare 3 He of Qingliangmi ［青粱米, Seed of Foxtail Millet, Setaria italica］ and grind it into powder. Prepare a handful of Chinese onion stalk.

上，煮作羹。下五味、椒、酱，空心食之。极治小便不通。

Make gruel with the above ingredients. Flavor with 5 kinds of seasonings, pepper, and sauce. Take on an empty stomach. It is effective to treat inhibited urination.

食治老人淋，烦热，小便茎中痛，涩少不快利。青豆方。

Qingdou Fang（Green Soya Bean Formula）is used to treat stranguria, heat with vexation, pain in the penis when urinating, and inhibited urine.

青豆二升　橘皮二两　麻子汁一升

Prepare 2 Sheng of green soy beans, 2 Liang of tangerine peel, and 1 Sheng of linseed decoction.

上，煮豆临熟，即下麻子汁。空心，渐食之，并服其汁皆验。

Boil the above ingredients, add linseed decoction when it is about to be cooked. Take the decoction slowly on an empty stomach.

食治老人五淋，久不止，身体壮热，小便满闷。小麦汤方。

Xiaomai Tang Fang（Wheat Soup Formula）is used to treat 5 types of persistent stranguria, vigorous heat, inhibited urine with symptoms of fullness and oppression of the aged.

小麦一升　通草二两

Prepare 1 Sheng of wheat and 2 Liang of Tongcao ［通草，Ricepaperplant Pith, Medulla Tetrapanacis］.

上，以水煮取三升，去滓。渐渐食之，须臾当差。

Boil the above ingredients, take 3 Sheng of the decoction and remove the dregs. Take it slowly and it will bring a rapid recovery.

食治老人淋病，小便长涩不利，痛闷之极。酥蜜煎方。

Sumi Jian Fang（Honey Decoction Formula）is used to treat stranguria, inhibited urine with symptoms of pain and oppression of the aged.

藕汁五合　白蜜五合　生地黄汁一升

Prepare 5 He of lotus root juice, 5 He of white honey, and 1 Sheng of Shengdihuang［生地黄, Unprocessed Rehmannia Root, Radix Rehmanniae Recens］juice.

上相和，微火煎之，令如饧。空心含半匙，渐渐下饮，食了亦服。忌热食炙肉。

Mix the above ingredients and decoct over low fire to make it look like maltose. Keep half a spoon of it in mouth on an empty stomach and drink it slowly. It is all right to take it after meal. It is contraindicated with hot food and roast meat.

食治老人五淋燥痛，小便不多，秘涩不通。苏粥方。

Suzhou Fang（Perilla Gruel Formula）is used to treat 5 types of stranguria, shortness of urine and inhibited urine of the aged.

土苏二两　青粱米四合，淘净　浆水二升

Prepare 2 Liang of Tusu［土苏, Perilla Leaf, Folium Perillae］and rinse 4 He of Qingliangmi［青粱米, Seed of Foxtail Millet, Setaria italica］. Prepare 2 Sheng of millet sour water.

上，煮作粥，临熟下苏搅之，空心食之，日一服尤佳。

Boil the above ingredients to make gruel. Add the perilla leaf when it is about to be cooked. Take on an empty stomach. It is effective to take it once a day.

食治老人淋病，小便下血，身体热盛。车前子饮。

Cheqianzi Yin（Plantain Seed Decoction）is used to treat stranguria, bloody urine and exuberant heat of the aged.

车前子五合，绵裹，水煮取汁　青粱米四合，淘研

Prepare 5 He of Cheqianzi［车前子, Plantain Seed, Semen Plantaginis］, wrap with cotton gauze and boil to get the juice. Wash 4 He of Qingliangmi［青粱米, Seed of Foxtail Millet, Setaria Italica］and grind it into powder.

上，煮煎汁作饮。空心食之。常服，亦明目，去热毒。

Boil and decoct the above ingredients. Take on an empty stomach. Long-term taking will brighten the eyes and eliminate heat-toxicity.

食治老人五淋秘涩，小便禁痛，膈闷不利。蒲桃浆方。

Putao Jiang Fang（Rose Apple Formula）is used to treat 5 types of stranguria, painful urination, and chest distress of the aged.

蒲桃汁一升　白蜜三合　藕汁一升

Prepare 1 Sheng of Putao ［蒲桃, Rose Apple, Syzygii Jamboris uFructus］ juice, 3 He of white honey, and 1 Sheng of lotus root juice.

上相和，微火温三沸即止。空心服五合，食后服五合。常以服之，殊效。

Mix the above ingredients together. Decoct on low fire for 3 times of boil. Take 5 He on an empty stomach and 5 He after meal. Long-term taking of it is effective.

增补方剂
Supplementary Formulas

食治老人热淋、石淋、尿急、尿频、少腹疼痛、小便黏稠有结块，或时下砂粒，舌苔白滑，脉沉弦者。白蒺藜茅根粥方。

Tribulusterrestris and Couch Grass Root Gruel Formula is used to treat stranguria due to heat or stone, urgent urination, frequent urination, lower abdominal pain, turbid urine or urine with granules for the aged with pale slippery tongue coating, deep and wiry pulse.

白蒺藜一两，包煎　　鲜茅根二两　　粳米一两，净淘

Prepare 1 Liang of Baijili ［白蒺藜, Tribulusribuli, Fructus］ wrapped with gauze, 2 Liang of Xianmaogen ［鲜茅根, Fresh Imperata Root, Imperatae Rhizoma Recens］, and 1 Liang of polished round-grained rice.

上三味，先煎白蒺藜鲜茅根，以水两碗熬取一碗半汁，过滤去滓，下粳米煮粥一碗，空心顿服之。日服二次，至病愈为度。

（经验方）

Decoct the former 2 ingredients first in 2 bowls of water until 1.5 bowls are left. Filter and remove the dregs. Add polished round-grained rice and make a bowl of gruel. Take it at a draught on an empty stomach twice a day until the disease is cured.

（Empirical Formula）

食治噎塞诸方

Formulas to Treat Dysphagia of the Aged with Diet Therapy

一

食治老人胸膈妨塞，食饮不下，渐黄瘦，行履无气，软弱。羊肉索饼方。

I

Yangrou Suobing Fang（Lamb Noodle Formula）is used to treat oppression in the chest and diaphragm, inability to take food, yellow complexion and emaciation, and flaccidity of the aged.

羊肉白者四两，切作臊头　　白面六两　　橘皮末一分

Prepare 4 Liang of Lamb and slice it to make condiment. Prepare 6 Liang of flour and 1 Fen of tangerine peel powder.

上，捣姜汁搜面。作之如常肉。下五味、葱、椒、姜、橘皮末等，炒熟煮。空心食之，日一服。极肥健脏腑。

Make noodles with the above ingredients and ginger juice. Cook it as usual. Flavor with 5 kinds of seasonings, green onion, pepper, ginger, tangerine peel powder, etc. Cook it thoroughly. Take on an empty stomach once a day. It is effective to strengthen the zang-fu organs.

二

食治老人噎病，心痛闷，膈气结，饮食不下。桂心粥方。

II

Guixin Zhou Fang（Cinnamon Bark Gruel Formula）is used to treat dysphagia, pain and oppression in the chest, qi stagnation in the diaphragm, and inability to take food of the aged.

桂心末一两　　粳米四合，淘研

Prepare 1 Liang of Guixin［桂心，Cinnamon Bark，Cortex Cinnamomi］powder. Prepare 4 He of polished round-grained rice, wash and grind into powder.

上，以煮作粥，半熟，次下桂末调和。空心日一服。亦破冷气殊效。

Cook gruel with the above ingredients. When it is half cooked, add cinnamon bark powder and mix it well. Take on an empty stomach once a day. It is also effective to eliminate cold qi.

食治老人噎病，食不通，胸胁满闷。黄雌鸡馎饦方。

Huangciji Botuo Fang（Yellow Hen Botuo Formula）is used to treat dysphagia, indigestion of food, fullness and distention in the chest and hypochondrium.

黄雌鸡四两，切作臛头　白面六两　茯苓末二两

Prepare 4 Liang of yellow chicken and slice it to make condiment, 6 Liang of flour, and 2 Liang of Fuling［茯苓, Indian Bread, Poria］powder.

上，和茯苓末，搜面作豉汁，中煮。空心食之。常作三五服，极除冷气噎。

Make dough with the above ingredients. Boil it in Douchi［豆豉, Fermented Soybean, Semen Sojae Preparatum］juice. Take on an empty stomach. It will take effect in relieving choking due to cold to take 3 or 5 doses regularly.

食治老人噎病，食饮不下，气塞不通。蜜浆方。

Mijiang Fang（Honey Beverage Formula）is used to treat dysphagia, inability to get food down and qi stagnation.

白蜜一两　熟汤一升

Prepare 1 Liang of white honey and 1 Sheng of cooked soup.

上,汤令熟,即下蜜调之。分二服,皆愈。

Boil the soup and mix it with honey. Take it in 2 doses and the disease will be cured.

食治老人噎病,气塞,食不通,吐逆。苏蜜煎方。

Sumi Jian Fang (Perilla and Honey Decoction Formula) is used to treat dysphagia, qi stagnation, indigestion of food, vomiting, and qi counter-flow of the aged.

土苏二两　白蜜五合　生姜汁五合

Prepare 2 Liang of Tusu [土苏, Perilla Leaf, Folium Perillae], 5 He of white honey, and 5 He of ginger juice.

上相和,微火煎之令沸。空心服半匙,细细下汁尤效。

Mix the above ingredients and decoct with low fire to bring to a boil. Take half a spoon on an empty stomach. It is very effective to swallow slowly.

食治老人噎病,胸满塞闷,饮食不下。姜橘汤方。

Jiangju Tang Fang (Ginger and Tangerine Decoction Formula) is used to treat dysphagia, fullness and distention in the chest, and inability to take food of the aged.

生姜二两，切　陈橘皮一两

Prepare 2 Liang of fresh ginger and slice, 1 Liang of Chenjupi〔陈橘皮, Dried Tangerine Peel, Pericarpium Citri Reticulatae〕.

上，以水二升，煎取一升，去滓，空心渐服之。常益。

Decoct the above ingredients with 2 Sheng of water until 1 Sheng of decoction is left. Remove the dregs and take on an empty stomach gradually. Long-term taking is good for health.

食治老人噎，脏腑虚弱，胸胁逆满，饮食不下。椒面粥方。

Jiaomian Zhou Fang (Pepper and Flour Gruel Formula) is used to treat dysphagia, weakness of the zang-fu organs, qi counter-flow and fullness in the chest and rib-side, inability to take food of the aged.

蜀椒一两，杵令碎　白面五两

Grind 1 Liang of Sichuan pepper into powder and prepare 5 Liang of flour.

上，以苦酒浸椒一宿，明旦取出，以拌面中，令匀，煮熟。空心食之。日二服，常验。

Soak the pepper in bitter wine for one night and take it out the next morning. Mix it in the flour thoroughly and cook it. Take on an empty stomach twice a day. It is very effective to take it often.

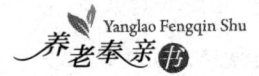

食治老人噎，冷气壅塞，虚弱，食不下。苏煎饼子。

Sujian Bingzi（Perilla Pancake Formula）is used to treat dysphagia, cold qi stagnation, flaccidity, and inability to take food of the aged.

土苏二两　白面六两，以生姜汁五合调之

Prepare 2 Liang of Tusu［土苏, Perilla Leaf, Folium Perillae］, 6 Liang of flour, mix them with 5 He of fresh ginger juice.

上，如常法作之。空心常食，润脏腑，和中。

Cook the above ingredients as usual and take on an empty stomach. Long-term taking will moisten the zang-fu organs and harmonize the middle energizer as well.

食治老人咽食入口，即塞涩不下，气壅。白米饮方。

Baimi Yin Fang（Rice Soup Formula）is used to treat inability to take food and qi congestion of the aged.

白米四合，研　舂头糠末一两

Prepare 4 He of rice and grind. Prepare 1 Liang of bran powder.

上，煮饮熟，下糠米调之。空心服食尤益。

Cook the above ingredients thoroughly. It is better to take on an empty stomach.

食治老人噎塞，水食不通，黄瘦羸弱。馄饨方。

Huntun Fang (Huntun Formula) is used to treat dysphagia, indigestion of food, emaciation with yellow complexion.

雌鸡肉五两，细切　　白面六两　　葱白半握

Prepare 5 Liang of hen and slice it thinly, 6 Liang of flour, and half a handful of scallion.

上，如常法，下五味、椒、姜向鸡汁中。煮熟空心食之。日一服，极补益。

Cook the above ingredients as usual. Add 5 kinds of seasonings, pepper and ginger. Take on an empty stomach once a day. It is very effective in nourishing and benefiting the body.

食治冷气诸方

Formulas to Treat Cold Syndrome of the Aged with Diet Therapy

一

食治老人冷气，心痛无时，往往发动，不能食。桃仁粥方。

I

Taoren Zhou Fang (Peach Seed Gruel Formula) is used to treat cold syndrome, irregular heartache, and inability to take food of the aged.

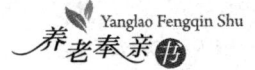

桃仁二两，去皮尖，研，水淘取　　青粱米四合，淘研

Prepare 2 Liang of peach seeds with the skin and pointed parts removed, 4 He of Qingliangmi［青粱米, Seed of Foxtail Millet, Setaria italica］and rinse clean.

上，以桃仁汁煮作粥，空心食之。常服，除冷温中。

Cook gruel with the above ingredients. Take on an empty stomach. Long-term taking will eliminate cold and warm the middle internal organs.

食治老人冷气，心痛不止，腹胀胁满，坐卧不得。茱萸饮方。

Zhuyu Yin Fang（Cornel Decoction Formula）is used to treat cold, endless heartache, abdominal distention and fullness, inability to sit or lie.

茱萸末二分　　青粱米二合，研细

Prepre 2 Fen of Zhuyu［茱萸, Medicinal Evodia Fruit powder, Fructus Evodiae］powder, 2 He of Qingliangmi［青粱米, Seed of Foxtail Millet, Setaria italica］and grind them finely.

上，以水二升，煎茱萸末，取一升，便下米煮作饮。空心食之，一二服尤佳。

Decoct the former with 2 Sheng of water until 1 Sheng decoction is left. Add rice and boil the decoction. Take on an empty stomach. It is better to take 1 or 2 doses.

二

食治老人冷气，心痛缴结，气闷。桂心酒方。

II

Guixin Jiu Fang（Cinnamon Bark Wine Formula）is used to treat cold syndrome, heart pain, unsmooth breath due to qi stagnation.

桂心末一两　清酒六合

Prepare 1 Liang of Guixin ［桂心, Cinnamon Bark, Cortex Cinnamomi］ powder and 6 He of rice wine.

上，温酒令热，即下桂心末调之。频服。一二服效。

Warm the wine, put the cinnamon bark powder in and mix them. Take it frequently. It will take effect after 1 to 2 doses.

食治老人冷气，心痛牵引背脊，不能下食。紫苏粥方。

Zisu Zhou Fang（Perilla Gruel Formula）is used to treat cold syndrome, heartache involving the back, inability to take food of the aged.

紫苏子三合，熬细，研　青粱米四合，淘

Prepare 3 He of Zisuzi ［紫苏子, Perilla Fruit, Perillae Fructus］, stew and grind fully. Prepare 4 He of Qingliangmi ［青粱米, Seed of Foxtail Millet, Setaria italica］ and rinse clean.

上，煮作粥，临熟下苏子末调之。空心服为佳。

Make gruel with the above ingredients. Add Zisuzi [紫苏子, Perilla Fruit, Perillae Fructus] powder when it is about to be cooked. It is better to take on an empty stomach.

食治老人冷气，卒心痛闷涩，气不来，手足冷。盐汤方。

Yantang Fang (Salt Soup Formula) is used to treat cold syndrome, acute heart pain, chest distress, shortness of breath, and cold limbs.

盐末一合　沸汤一升

Prepare 1 He of salt and 1 Sheng of boiled soup.

上以盐末内汤中，调。频令服尽。须臾当吐。吐即差。

Add salt to the soup and stir them. Take it frequently to induce vomiting, then the disease will be cured.

食治老人冷气心痛，呕不多，下食烦闷。椒面馎饦方。

Jiaomian Botuo Fang (Pepper Botuo Formula) is used to treat the aged with cold syndrome, heartache, slight vomiting, vexation and oppression after taking meals.

蜀椒一两，去目及闭口者，焙干为末，筛　白面五两　葱白三茎，切

Prepare 1 Liang of uncracked Sichuan pepper, remove the pit, dry by the fire, grind into powder, and sieve it. Prepare 5 Liang of flour, 3 pieces of Chinese onion white and slice.

上，以椒末和面，搜作之，水煮。下五味调和食之，常三五服极效，尤佳。

Make dough with the above ingredients and boil. Flavor it with 5 kinds of seasonings. It is very effective to take 3 to 5 doses regularly.

食治老人冷气心痛。姜橘皮汤方。

Jiangjupi Tang Fang（Ginger and Tangerine Peel Soup Formula）is used to treat the aged with cold syndrome and pain in heart.

生姜一两，切　陈橘皮一两，炙，为末

Prepare 1 Liang of fresh ginger sliced and 1 Liang of Chenjupi ［陈橘皮，Dried Tangerine Peel, Pericarpium Citri Reticulatae］ roasted into powder.

上以水一升，煎取七合，去滓，空心食之，日三两服尤益。

Boil the above ingredients in 1 Sheng of water and decoct until 7 He decoction is left. Remove the dregs and take on an empty stomach. It is very effective to take 2 to 3 doses one day.

食治老人冷气，心痛郁结，两胁胀满。高良姜粥方。

Gaoliangjiang Zhou Fang（Lesser Galangal Rhizome Gruel Formula）is used to treat cold syndrome, heart pain, binding depression, distention and fullness in the ribs of the aged.

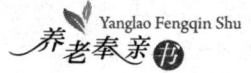

高良姜二两，切，以水二升，煎取一升半汁　青粱米四合，研淘

Prepare 2 Liang of Gaoliangjiang［高良姜, Lesser Galangal Rhizome, Rhizoma Alpiniae Officinarum］, slice and decoct it in 2 Sheng of water until 1.5 Sheng decoction is left. Prepare 4 He of Qingliangmi［青粱米, Seed of Foxtail Millet, Setaria italica］and rinse clean.

上，以姜汁煮粥。空心食之。日一服，极益效。

Make gruel with the above ingredients. Take on an empty stomach once a day. It is very effective to cure the disease.

食治老人冷气，心痛发动，时遇冷风即痛。荜茇粥方。

Biba Zhou Fang（Long Pepper Gruel Formula）is used to treat cold syndrome, heart pain, and pain due to cold wind of the aged.

荜茇末，二合　胡椒末，一分　青粱米四合, 淘

Prepare 2 He of long pepper powder, 1 Fen of pepper powder, and 4 He of Qingliangmi［青粱米, Seed of Foxtail Millet, Setaria italica］and rinse clean.

上，以煮作粥，熟，下二味调之。空心食。常服尤效。

Cook gruel with the millet and flavor with the former 2 ingredients when the gruel is cooked. Take on an empty stomach. Long-term taking is good for health.

食治老人冷气逆，心痛结，举动不得。干姜酒方。

Ganjiang Jiu Fang（Dried Ginger Wine Formula）is used to treat cold syndrome, counter-flow of qi, heart pain and binding, and inability to move of the aged.

干姜末，半两　清酒六合

Prepare Half Liang of dried ginger powder and 6 He of rice wine.

上，温酒热，即下椒末投酒中。顿服之，立愈。

Warm the wine and put pepper powder in it. Take at a draught and a rapid recovery will be attained.

增补方剂

Supplementary Formulas

食治老人血虚，冷气内侵，腹中拘急，绵绵作痛，喜得温按，及寒疝腹中痛，胁痛里急者。当归生姜羊肉汤方。

Angelica, ginger and lamb soup formula can be used to treat blood deficiency, invasion of cold to the internal, contracture and continuous pain in the abdomen which prefers warmth and pressure, abdomenal pain due to cold hernia, and hypochondriac pain of the aged.

当归三两　生姜五两　羊肉一斤

Prepare 3 Liang of Danggui [当归, Chinese Angelica, Radix Angelicae Sinensis], 5 Liang of fresh ginger, and 1 Jin of lamb.

上三味，以水八升，煮取三升，温服七合，日三服。若寒多者加生姜成一斤；痛多而呕者加橘皮二两，白术一两。加生姜者亦加水五升，煮取三升二合，服之。

（《金匮要略》）

Decoct the above ingredients in 8 Sheng of water until 3 Sheng soup is left. Take 7 He when it is warm 3 times a day. For patients with heavier cold syndrome, 1 Jin of fresh ginger can be used. For patients with pain and vomiting, 2 Liang of tangerine peel and 1 Liang of Baizhu [白术, Argehead Atractylodes Rhizome, Rhizoma Atractylodis Macrocephalae] can be used. At this time, add 5 Sheng of water and decoct until 3 Sheng and 2 He soup is left.

Jin Gui Yao Lue（*Synopsis of the Golden Chamber*）

食治诸痔方

Formulas to Treat Hemorrhoids of the Aged with Diet Therapy

食治老人痔病，下血不止，肛门肿。猫狸羹方。

Limao Geng Fang（Leopard Cat Soup Formula）is used to treat hemorrhoid with incessant bleeding and anal swelling of the aged.

猫狸一两，如常法治

Prepare 1 Liang of leopard cat meat. Clean it as usual.

上细切，以面及葱、椒、五味拌，作片炙熟。空心，渐食之。亦可作羹粥，任性尤佳。

Slice the meat thinly, flavor with flour, Chinese onion, pepper, and 5 kinds of seasonings, roast it. Take it slowly on an empty stomach. It can also be made into gruel and take as one likes.

食治老人痔，下血久不差，渐加黄瘦，无力。鲤鱼鲙方。

Liyu Kuai Fang（Sliced Carp Formula）is used to treat hemorrhoid with continuous bleeding, yellow complexion, emaciation and flaccidity.

鲤鱼肉十两，切作鲙，如常法

Prepare 10 Liang of carp and slice as usual.

上以蒜、醋、五味，空心常食之，日一服，极差。忌鲊、甜食。

Flavor the above ingredients with garlic, vinegar and 5 kinds of seasonings. Take it regularly on an empty stomach. It will take effect after one dose a day. It is contraindicated with salted fish and sweet food.

食治老人痔，常下血，身体壮热，不多食。苍耳粥方。

Cang'er Zhou Fang（Xanthium Gruel Formula）is used to treat hemorrhoid with frequent bleeding, vigorous heat and poor appetite of the aged.

苍耳子五合，熟，拌水二升，煎取一升半汁　粳米四合，淘

Prepare 5 He of Cang'erzi［苍耳子, Xanthium, Xanthii Fructus］. Decoct it in 2 Sheng of water until 1.5 Sheng is left. Rinse 1 He of polished round-grained rice.

上，以前件煮作粥。空心食之。日常服，亦可煎汤服之，极效。破气明目。

Cook gruel with the above ingredients. Take it regularly on an empty stomach, It can also be taken as soup. It is very effective to break qi stagnation and improve the eyesight.

食治老人痔，病久不愈，肛门肿痛。鳗鲡鱼臛方。

Manliyu Huo Fang（Eel Broth Formula）is used to treat lingering hemorrhoid and swelling and pain of the anus of the aged.

鳗鲡鱼肉一斤，切作臛　葱白半握，细切

Prepare 1 Jin of eel meat and slice it to make broth. Prepare half a handful of scallion and slice it thinly.

上，煮作臛下五味、椒、姜。空心渐食之。杀虫尤佳。

Boil the above ingredients and flavor with 5 kinds of seasonings, pepper and ginger to make meat sauce. Take it slowly on an empty stomach. It is very effective to kill roundworm.

食治老人痔病下血不止，日加羸瘦无力。鸲鹆散方。

Quyu San Fang (Crested Myna Powder Formula) is used to treat hemorrhoid with incessant bleeding, emaciation and lack of strength of the aged.

鸲鹆五只，治洗令净，曝令干

Prepare 5 crested mynas, process and wash clean, dry them in the sun.

上，捣为散。空心，以白粥饮，服二方寸匕，日二服，最验。亦可炙食任性。

Grind the above ingredients into powder. Take 2 square-inch-spoons of it twice a day with plain rice porridge on an empty stomach. It can also be roasted and taken as much as one likes.

食治老人五痔，泄血不绝，四肢衰弱，不能下食。杏仁饮方。

Xingren Yin Fang (Apricot Kernel Decoction Formula) is used to treat 5 kinds of hemorrhoids with incessant bleeding, weak limbs and inability to take food of the aged.

杏仁二两，去皮尖，细研，以水浸之　粳米四合，淘之

Prepare 2 Liang of Xingren [杏仁, Bitter Apricot Seed, Semen Armeniacae Amarum] with the skin and pointed parts removed, grind and soak in water. Prepare 4 He of polished round-grained rice and rinse clean.

上，以杏仁汁相和，煮作饮。空心食之，日一服效。

Mix and boil the above ingredients with apricot kernel juice. Take on an empty stomach once a day.

食治老人五痔久不愈，生疮疼痛。野猪肉羹方。

Yezhurou Geng Fang（Wild Boar Meat Sauce Formula）is used to treat 5 kinds of lingering hemorrhoids, sores and pains of the aged.

野猪肉一斤，细切　葱白一握　米二合，细研

It is composed of 1 Jin of thinly-sliced wild boar meat, a handful of Chinese onion stalk and 2 He of thoroughly ground rice.

上，煮作羹。五味调和椒姜，空心渐食之。常作极效。

Make gruel with the above ingredients. Flavor with the 5 kinds of seasonings, pepper, and ginger. Take it slowly on an empty stomach. Long-term taking is good for health.

食治老人五痔下血，常烦热，羸瘦。桑耳粥方。

Sanger Zhou Fang（Mulberry Wood Ear Gruel Formula）is used to treat 5 kinds of hemorrhoids with bleeding, frequent heat with vexation and emaciation of the aged.

桑耳二两，水三升，煎取二升汁　粳米四合，淘之

Boil 2 Liang of Sang'er［桑耳, Mulberry Wood Ear, Mori Auricularia

Auricula] in 3 Sheng of water until 2 Sheng remains. Prepare 4 He of polished round-grained rice and rinse clean.

上，以桑耳汁煮，作粥，空心食之，日一二服，皆效。
Cook gruel with the above ingredients. Take on an empty stomach. It is effective to take 1 or 2 doses a day.

食治老人五痔，泄血不止，积日困劣无气。鸳鸯法炙方。
Yuanyang Fazhi Fang (Roast Mandarin Duck Formula) is used to treat 5 kinds of hemorrhoids with incessant bleeding, daytime drowsiness due to shortness of qi of the aged.

鸳鸯一枚，如常法
Prepare and clean 1 Yuanyang [鸳鸯 , Mandarin Duck, Aicis Caro] as usual.

上，以五味、椒、酱腌，火炙之，令熟。空心渐食之。亦疗久瘘疮绝验。
Flavor with 5 kinds of seasonings, pepper, and sauce. Then roast on the fire to cook it. Take it slowly on an empty stomach. It is also very effective to treat enduring fistula and sore.

食治老人五痔，血下不差，肛门肿痛，渐瘦。鲇鱼方。
Nianyu Fang (Catfish Formula) is used to treat 5 kinds of hemorrhoids with bleeding, swelling and pain of the anus and gradual emaciation of the

aged.

鲇鱼肉一斤　葱白半把

Prepare 1 Jin of catfish and half a handful of Chinese onion stalk.

上，以白煮令熟，空心，以蒜、醋、五味，渐渐食之，常作尤佳。

Boil the above ingredients in water. Flavor with garlic, vinegar, and 5 kinds of seasonings. Take it slowly on an empty stomach. Long-term taking of it is effective.

增补方剂

Supplementary Formulas

老人痔疮下血久不止，或自溃出脓血，痔核肿痛，虚羸自汗，右脉虚大无力者。黄芪粥方主之。

Milkvetch Root Gruel Formula is used to treat hemorrhoid with persistent bleeding, or ulcerated pus and blood, swelling and sore caused by hemorrhoid, spontaneous sweating due to deficiency and emaciation for the aged with deficient and weak pulse on the right.

黄芪一两，细切　刺猬皮五钱，炙　粳米二两，淘净

Prepare 1 Liang of Huangqi［黄芪，Milkvetch Root, Radix Astragali seu Hedysari］ and slice thinly. Roast 5 Qian of hedgehog skin. Wash 2 Liang of polished round-grained rice.

上，以水两大碗，先煎黄芪、刺猬皮至一碗半，去滓，下米煮粥，空腹食之，每日一次。

（经验方）

Decoct the former 2 ingredients with 2 bowls of water until 1.5 bowl is left. Remove the dregs and add rice to make gruel. Take on an empty stomach once a day.

（Empirical Formula）

食治诸风方

Formulas to Treat Wind Syndrome of the Aged with Diet Therapy

食治老人中风，言语謇涩，精神昏愦，手足不仁，缓弱不遂方。

Huanruo Busui Fang（Paralysis Relieving Formula）is used to treat wind stroke, sluggish speech, dotage, and numbness in the limbs of the aged.

葛粉五两　荆芥一握　豉五合

It is composed of 5 Liang of Gefen〔葛粉，Pueraria Starch, Puerariae Amylum〕, a handful of Jingjie〔荆芥，Fineleaf Schizonepeta Herb, Herba Schizonepetae〕, and 5 He of Douchi〔豆豉，Fermented Soybean, Semen Sojae Preparatum〕.

上，以搜葛粉，如常作之，煎二味取汁煮之，下葱、椒、五味、腥头，

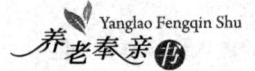

空心食之一二服，将息为效。忌猪肉荞面。

Mix with Gefen［葛粉，Pueraria Starch, Puerariae Amylum］and cook as usual. Add the other ingredients, decoct and flavor with Chinese onion, pepper, 5 kinds of seasonings, and condiment. Take 1 or 2 doses on an empty stomach. A good rest will make it more effective. It is contraindicated with pork and buckwheat.

食治老人中风，口面㖞偏，大小便秘涩，烦热。荆芥粥方。

Jinjie Zhou Fang（Schizonepeta Gruel Formula）is used to treat wind stroke with deviated mouth and face, constipation, rough urination, and heat with vexation of the aged.

荆芥一把，切　青粱米四合，淘　薄荷叶半握，切　豉五合，绵裹

Prepare a handful of Jingjie［荆芥，Fineleaf Schizonepeta Herb, Herba Schizonepetae］and slice. Wash 4 He of Qingliangmi［青粱米，Seed of Foxtail Millet, Setaria italica］. Prepare half a handful of Bohe［薄荷，Peppermint, Herba Menthae］and slice, 5 He of Douchi［豆豉，Fermented Soybean, Semen Sojae Preparatum］and make it cotton-wrapped.

上，以水煮取荆芥汁，下米及诸味，煮作粥，入少盐、醋。空心食之。常服佳。

Boil the first ingredient to get the juice, then add rice and flavors to make gruel, flavor with a little salt and vinegar. Take on an empty stomach. Long-term taking is good for health.

食治老人中风，缓弱不仁，四肢摇动，无气力。炙熊肉方。

Zhi Xiongrou Fang (Roast Bear Formula) is used to treat wind stroke, numbness and shaking of the limbs, and lack of strength.

熊肉一斤，切　葱白半握，切　酱椒等

It is composed of 1 Jin of sliced bear meat, half a handful of Chinese onion stalk sliced thinly, pepper sauce, etc.

上，以五味腌之。炙熟，空心冷食之。恒服为佳。亦可作羹粥，任性食之尤佳。

Pickle the above ingredients with 5 kinds of seasonings. Roast them and take on an empty stomach. Long-term taking is good for health. It can also be taken as gruel and it is better to take as much as one likes.

食治老人中风汗出，四肢顽痹，言语不利。麻子饮方。

Mazi Yin Fang (Hemp Seed Decoction Formula) is used to treat wind stroke, sweating, impediment of the limbs and sluggish speech of the aged.

麻子五合，熬，细研，水淹取汁　粳米四合，净淘，研之

Boil 5 He of hemp seed, grind thoroughly, soak in water and take the decoction. Wash 4 He of polished round-grained rice and grind it.

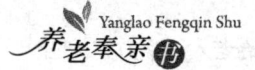

上以麻子煮作饮，空心渐食之，频作极补益。

Boil the above ingredients and take it on an empty stomach slowly. It nourishes and benefits the body greatly if taken frequently.

食治老人中风，口目眴动，烦闷不安。牛蒡馎饦方。

Niubang Botuo Fang (Burdock Botuo Formula) is used to treat wind stroke, twitching of the mouth and eyes, vexation and agitation of the aged.

牛蒡根切一升，去皮，曝干，杵为面　白米四合，净淘研之

Prepare 1 Sheng of Niubanggen [牛蒡根, Arctium Root, Arctii Radix] and peel. Dry in the sun and grind into powder. Prepare 4 He of rice and rinse.

上，以牛蒡粉和面作之，向豉汁中煮。加葱、椒、五味、臛头，空心食之。恒服极效。

Make dough with burdock powder and boil in Douchi [豆豉, Fermented Soybean, Semen Sojae Preparatum] juice. Flavor with Chinese onions, pepper, 5 kinds of seasonings, and condiment. Take on an empty stomach. Long-term taking will be very effective.

食治老人卒中风，口噤，身体反张，不语。大豆酒方。

Dadou Jiu Fang (Soybean Wine Formula) is used to treat wind stroke, lockjaw, arched-back rigidity, and speechlessness of the aged.

大豆二升，熬之　　清酒二升

Boil 2 Sheng of soybeans and prepare 2 Sheng of rice wine.

上，熬豆令声绝，即下酒投之，煮一二沸，去滓。顿服之。覆卧取汗，差。口噤，拗灌之。

Boil the beans thoroughly and pour the wine in, bring it to 1 or 2 boils. Remove the dregs. Take it at a draught and then lie to promote sweating with coverings on. The disease will be cured. Force the patient with lockjaw to open the mouth and take medicine.

食治老人中风，头旋目眩，身体厥强，筋骨疼痛，手足烦热，心神不安。乌驴头方。

Wulütou Fang（Black Donkey Head Formula）is used to treat wind stroke, dizziness, stiff body, pain in the sinews and bones, feverish sensation in limbs, and malaise of the aged.

乌驴头一枚，炮，去毛净治

Prepare one black donkey head, process it and remove the hair and wash clean.

上，以煮令烂熟，细切。空心，以姜、醋、五味食之。渐进为佳。极除风热，其汁如酽酒，亦医前患尤效。

Cook it thoroughly and slice thinly. Flavor with ginger, vinegar, and 5 kinds of seasonings. Take it slowly on an empty stomach. It is very effective to dispel wind-heat. Its decoction looks like thick wine, which is also effective to treat the disease.

食治老人中风，四肢不仁，筋骨顽强。苍耳叶羹方。
Cang'er ye Geng Fang（Cocklebur Leaf Formula）is used to treat wind stroke, numbness of the limbs, and strengthen the sinew and bone of the aged.

苍耳叶五两，切好嫩者　　豉心二两，别煎
Slice 5 Liang of tender cocklebur leaf. Decoct 2 Liang of Douchi［豆豉, Fermented Soybean, Semen Sojae Preparatum］separately.

上，和煮作羹。下五味、椒、姜调和，空心食之尤佳。
Make soup with the above ingredients. Flavor with 5 kinds of seasonings, pepper, and ginger. Take on an empty stomach.

食治老人中风，热毒，心闷，气壅昏倒。甘草豆方。
Gancaodou Fang（Liquorice and Black Bean Formula）is used to treat wind stroke, heat-toxicity, oppression in the chest, faint due to qi stagnation.

甘草一两　　乌豆三合　　生姜半两，切
It is composed of 1 Liang of Gancao［甘草, Liquorice Root, Glycyrrhiza

Uralensis Fisch.〕, 3 He of black beans and half Liang of sliced ginger.

上，以水二升，煎取一升，去滓。冷，渐食服之。极治热毒。

Boil the above ingredients in 2 Sheng of water until 1 Sheng is left. And remove the dregs Take it slowly when it cools down. It is very effective to treat heat-toxicity.

食治老人中风烦热，言语涩闷，手足热。乌鸡臛方。

Wuji Huo Fang（Black Chicken Broth Formula）is used to treat wind stroke, heat with vexation, sluggish speech, fever of the hands and feet.

乌鸡半斤，细切　麻子汁五合　葱白一把

Slice half Jin of black chicken thinly. Prepare 5 He of sesame seed juice and a handful of scallion.

上，煮作臛，次下麻汁、五味、椒姜令熟。空心渐食之。补益。

Cook the black chicken into broth, then put in the sesame seed juice, 5 kinds of seasonings, pepper and ginger. Take it slowly on an empty stomach. It nourishes and benefits the body.

食治老人中风，心神昏昧，行即欲倒，呕吐。白羊头方。

Baiyangtou Fang（White Lamb Head Formula）is used to treat wind stroke, confusion of consciousness, susceptibility to fall down when walking, and vomiting of the aged.

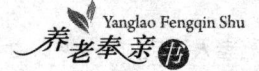

白羊头一具，治如常法

Prepare 1 white lamb head and boil it as usual.

上，以空心，用姜醋渐食之为佳。

Flavor it with ginger and vinegar, and take it slowly on an empty stomach.

食治老人中风邪毒，脏腑壅塞，手足缓弱，蒜煎。

Suan Jian (Garlic Decoction Formula) is used to treat wind stroke, pathogenic toxin, stagnation of the zang-fu organs, flaccidity of the limbs of the aged.

大蒜一升，去皮，细切　大豆黄炒二升

Prepare 1 Sheng of garlic, peel and slice thinly. Fry 2 Jin of soybeans.

上，以水一升，和二味，微火煎之，似稠即止。空心，每服食啖三二匙。亦补肾气。

Decoct the above ingredients in 1 Sheng of water on low fire till it is thick. Take 2 or 3 spoons for each dose on an empty stomach. It can also be used to tonify the kidney qi.

食治老人久风湿痹，筋挛骨痛。润皮毛，益气力，补虚，止毒，除面䵟。宜服补肾地黄酒。

Bushen Dihuang Jiu (Rehmannia Wine Formula with Kidney-tonifying Function) is used to treat rheumatism due to wind and dampness, spasm of the sinews, and pain of the bones of the aged. It can moisten the skin and hair, replenish qi and strength, restore deficiency, eliminate toxin, improve dull and dark complexion.

生地黄一斤，切　大豆二升，熬之　生牛蒡根一升，切

It is composed of 1 Jin of sliced Shengdihuang〔生地黄, Unprocessed Rehmannia Root, Radix Rehmanniae Recens〕, 2 Sheng of soybeans that are boiled, and 1 Sheng of sliced Shengniubang〔生牛蒡, arctium, Arctii Fructus〕.

上，以绢袋盛之，以酒一斗，浸之五六日。任性空心温服。常服三二盏。恒作之尤佳。

Put the above ingredients into a silk bag and then soak in 1 Dou of wine for 5 to 6 days. Warm and take 2 to 3 small cups each time on an empty stomach. Long-term taking is very effective.

食治老人风，热烦毒，顽痹不仁，五缓六急。驼脂酒方。

Tuozhi Jiu Fang (Camel Fat Wine Formula) is used to treat wind disease, heat with vexation, impediment and numbness due to wind, cold and dampness of the aged.

野驼脂五两，炼之为上

It is composed of 5 Liang of wild camel fat. The refined one is of high quality.

上，空心温酒五合下半匙以上，调脂令消，顿服之，日二服，极效。

Warm 5 He of wine and add more than half a spoon of the above ingredient. Stir to make the fat dissolve. Take at a draught twice a day. It is very effective to treat the disease.

食治老人风挛拘急，偏枯不通利。雁脂酒方。

Yanzhi Jiu Fang（Wild Goose Fat Wine Formula）is used to treat spasm and contraction of tendons, and hemiplegia of the aged.

雁脂五两，消之令散

Prepare 5 Liang of wild goose fat and cook until it melts.

上，每日空心温酒一盏，下脂半合许调，顿服之。

Mix a cup of warm wine and half He of fat together. Take at a draught on an empty stomach every day.

食治老人风虚痹弱，四肢无力，腰膝疼痛。巨胜酒方。

Jusheng Jiu Fang（Black Sesame Wine Formula）is used to treat weakness and impediment due to wind deficiency, flaccidity of the limbs, and pain in the lumbus and knees of the aged.

巨胜子二斤，熬　薏苡仁二升　干地黄半斤，切

It is composed of 2 Jin of black sesames that are boiled, 2 Sheng of

Yiyiren［薏苡仁, Coix, Semen Coicis］, and half Jin of sliced Gandihuang［干地黄, Dried Rehmannia, Rehmanniae Radix］.

上，以绢袋贮，无灰酒一斗渍之，勿令泄气。满五六日，任性空心温服一二盏尤益。

Put the above ingredients into a silk bag, soak in 1 Dou of lime-free rice wine and seal closely. After 5 to 6 days, warm it and take 1 or 2 small cups on an empty stomach as one likes.

食治老人风冷痹，筋脉缓急。苍耳茶方。

Cang'er Cha Fang（Cocklebur Fruit Tea Formula）is used to treat impediment due to wind and cold, and spasm and stiffness of the sinews of the aged.

苍耳子二升，熬杵为末

Boil 2 Sheng of Cang'erzi［苍耳子, Siberian Cocklebur Fruit, Fructus Xanthii］and smash it into powder.

上，每日煎服之。代茶常服，治风热明目。

Decoct and drink it as tea every day. It is very effective to treat wind-heat and brighten the eyesight.

食治老人热风下血，明目，益气除邪，治齿疼，利脏腑顺气。槐茶方。

Huaicha Fang（Sophora Leaf Tea Formula）is used to treat bloody stool due to heat wind, brighten the eyesight, replenish qi, eliminate pathogenic factors, treat toothache, benefit the zang-fu organs, and promote qi circulation of the aged.

槐叶嫩者五斤，蒸令熟，为片，曝干作茶，捣罗为末

Steam 5 Jin of tender sophora leaves and cut them into slices. Dry in the sun and grind into powder.

上，每日煎如茶法，服之恒益，除风尤佳。

Decoct the powder and drink it as tea for a long time. It is very effective to eliminate wind pathogen.

简妙老人备急方
Simple and Effective Formulas for Emergency of the Aged

治一切损血出，消肿毒。秦王背指散。

Qinwang Beizhi San（The King of Qin's Dorsal Finger Powder）can treat various bleeding caused by wounds, subside swelling, and remove toxin.

宣连 槟榔各等分

Prepare Xuanlian ［宣连，Golden Thread, Rhizoma Coptidis］ and Binglang ［槟榔，Areca Seed, Semen Arecae］ in equal amount.

上为末，伤扑干贴，消肿冷水调鸡翎扫，妙。

Pound the above ingredients into powder. Put it on the wound to dry, or mix it with cold water and apply on the swelling part with chicken feather.

治失音。回声饮子。
Huisheng Yinzi（Voice Recovering Decoction）can treat loss of voice.

皂角一挺，刮去黑皮并子　萝卜二个，切作片
Prepare one Zaojiao ［皂角，Chinese Honeylocust Fruit, Spina Gleditsiae］ with its dark skin and seeds removed. Cut 2 Chinese radishes into pieces.

上以水二碗，同煎至半碗以下，服之不过三服，便语。吃却萝卜更妙。
Decoct the above ingredients in 2 bowls of water until half bowl of water is left. The voice will be recovered after taking 3 doses. And it will have better effect if taking Chinese radish at the same time.

治鼻衄。醍醐酒。
Tihu Jiu（Wine Made of Clarified Butter）is used to treat epistaxis.

上以萝卜自然汁半盏，热酒半盏，相和令匀，再用汤温过，服之立验。
Blend half cup of fresh radish juice with half cup of hot wine, warm the mixture and take it. The epistaxis will be cured immediately.

补下元，乌髭须，壮脚膝，进食，悦颜色，治腰疼。杜仲丸。
Duzhong Wan（Eucommia Bark Pill）is used to black hair, strengthen

the feet and knees, improve appetite, boost mood, and treat lumbago by tonifying the kidney qi.

杜仲一两，炙令黄为度　补骨脂一两，炒令香熟，为末　胡桃仁一两，汤浸去皮，细研

Prepare one Liang of Duzhong［杜仲，Eucommia, Cortex Eucommiae］stir-fried to brown, one Liang of Buguzhi［补骨脂，Psoralea, Fructus Psoraleae］stir-fried and cooked into powder, and one Liang of Taoren［桃仁，Peach Seed, Semen Perisicae］soaked in hot water to remove the skin and ground into powder.

上件三味，研令匀，炼蜜为丸如梧桐子大。空心，温酒下三十丸。

Pound the 3 ingredients into powder, and make them into pills with refined honey as big as firmiana seeds. Take 30 pills with warm wine on an empty stomach.

治一切眼，洗眼药。

Xiyan Yao（Eye-washing Lotion）can treat all kinds of eye disorders.

胆矾一两，煅令白，去火毒用　滑石一两，研　秦皮半两　腻粉二钱匕

Prepare one Liang of Danfan［胆矾，Chalcanthite, Chalcanthitum］forged to white to remove its fire toxin, one Liang of Huashi［滑石，Talcum, Pulvis Talci］grounded into powder, half a Liang of Qinpi［秦皮，Ash Bark,

Cortex Fraxini〕, and 4 Qian and 7 Fen of Nifen〔腻粉, Calomel, Calomelas Calomel〕.

上每用一字，汤泡候温，闭目洗两眦头，以冷为度。

Take a spoon of each above mentioned ingredients, soak them in hot water and wait until it is warm, close eyes and wash the canthi with the lotion until it is cold.

补益，疗眼有黑花。明目川椒丸。

Mingmu Chuanjiao Wan（Eyesight Improving Pricklyash Peel Pill）is a tonic that can treat blurred vision.

川椒一斤，每用盐一斤，拌淹一宿，三度换盐，淹三夜，取出晒干，去盐用　黑参半斤，锉

Prepare one Jin of Chuanjiao〔川椒, Pricklyash Peel, Pericarpium Zanthoxyli〕, submerge it in one Jin of salt for 3 nights, change the salt 3 times for each night, take it out and dry in the sun, desalt before use. Prepare half a Jin of Heishen〔黑参, Black Ginseng, Scrophularia ningpoensis Hemsl〕filed.

上二味为末，炼蜜为丸如梧桐子大。每日盐汤下三十丸，食后临卧服之。

Pound the above ingredients into powder, and make them into pills with refined honey as big as firmiana seeds. Take 30 pills each day with salt soup after meal before going to bed.

治肾脏虚冷，肝膈浮热上冲，两目生翳黑花，风毒久不治者。

This formula① can treat blurred vision and chronic wind toxin due to asthenic cold in the kidney, and heat counter-flow of the liver and diaphragm.

青盐一两，生研　苍术一两，先用米泔水浸洗三日，焙干，切　木贼草一两，小便浸三日，焙干

Prepare one Liang of raw Qingyan ［青盐，Halite, Halitum］ grounded, one Liang of Cangzhu ［苍术，Rhizoma Atractylodis, Rhizoma Atractylodis］ sliced and baked after being soaked in rice water for 3 days, and one Liang of Muzeicao ［木贼草，Horsetail, Equisetum hyemale L.］ baked after being soaked in urine for 3 days.

上为末，空心熟水调下一钱。如大段青白不见物者，不过十服。小可，只二三服。

Pound the above ingredients into powder, take one Qian of it with boiled water on an empty stomach. For blindness with blurred bluish white, it can be cured with 10 doses. For mild eye disorder, it can be cured with 2 or 3 doses.

---

① 根据校注，该方为盐术木贼散〔Salt, Atractylodes Rhizome and Horsetail Powder）.

治眼有冷泪。木贼散。

Muzei San（Horsetail Powder）can treat epiphora induced by wind.

木贼一两，为末　木耳一两，烧为黑灰

Prepare one Liang of Muzeicao［木贼草, Horsetail, Equisetum hyemale L.］ground into powder, 1 Liang of Muer［木耳, Dried Fungus, Auricularia Auricula］burned into black ashes.

上件二味，同研令匀。每用二钱，以清米泔煎熟，放温调下。食后，临卧各一服。

Pound the 2 ingredients into powder, decoct 2 Qian of it with clear rice water each time. Take one dose after meal and one before sleep.

治肠风泻血当日止方：

Hemostasis formula can take instant effect in dealing with hemafecia due to intestinal wind.

附子一两,炮去皮、脐,为末　绿矾四两,用瓶子盛之,火煅食,顷候冷取,入盐一合,硫黄一两,同矾研,依前入瓶子内烧食,久候冷取出，研细用之

Prepare 1 Liang of Fuzi［附子, Prepared Common Monkshood Daughter Root, Radix Aconiti Lateralis Preparata］, process and ground it into powder with its skin and navel removed. Prepare 4 Liang of Lüfan［绿矾, Melanterite, Melanteritum］, store it in the bottle, forge and wait until it is cold, mix in 1 He of salt and 1 Liang of sulfur, pestle and put them in the bottle to forge again, take them out after they are cold, then pound them into powder.

上二味，一处研令匀，粟米粥为丸，如梧桐子大。空心，用生地黄汁下三十丸，当日止。一月除根，亦可久服。助下元，除风气，补益脏腑。

Grind the above 2 ingredients and mix with millet gruel, make them into pills as big as firmiana seeds. Take 30 pills with the juice of Shengdihuang [生地黄, Unprocessed Rehmannia Root, Radix Rehmanniae Recens] on an empty stomach and the bleeding would be stopped the same day. After taking it for one month, the disease can be cured, and it can also be taken for a long time for better effect. It can strengthen the kidney qi, expel the wind pathogen, and nourish the zang-fu organs.

治泻痢。乳香散。和气，止脏毒泻血，腹内疼痛等。

Ruxiang San (Olibanum Powder) can treat diarrhea, harmonize qi, stop bloody diarrhea due to toxin in the zang-organs, and relieve the abdominal pain.

乳香少许　诃子皮一分　当归半两　木香半分

Prepare a little Ruxiang [乳香, Olibanum, Resina Olibani], a Fen of the peel of Hezi [诃子, Terminalia, Fructus Chebulae], half a Liang of Danggui [当归, Angelica, Radix Angelicae Sinensis], and half a Fen of Muxiang [木香, Costusroot, Radix Aucklandiae].

上细锉，与乳香微炒，候当归干为度，杵为末。每服二钱，用陈米第三度泔，六分一盏，煎至五分。空心，午前服。此方最妙，患及百余日者，服之皆愈。

Grind the ingredients and fry them slightly with Ruxiang［乳香，Olibanum, Resina Olibani］, pound them into powder when Danggui［当归，Angelica, Radix Angelicae Sinensis］ is dried. Take 2 Qian each time, use the third-time washing water of stale rice, put it in the cup with 6 Fen of water, decoct until five sixths is left. Take it before noon on an empty stomach. This formula is very effective and can cure the disorder lasting as long as 100 days.

芸香丸。治风血留滞，下成肠风痔疾。

Yunxiang Wan（Bird Rape Pill）can treat intestinal wind and hemorrhoid due to blood stasis.

鹿角一两，烧令红，候冷研　芸薹子半两，微炒

Prepare one Liang of Lujiao［鹿角，Deerhorn, Cervus Elaphus Linnaeus］ burned to red and ground into powder after cooling down, half a Liang of Yuntaizi［芸薹子，Seeds of Bird Rape, Semen Brassicae Campestris］ stir-fried slightly.

上二味为末，醋煮面糊为丸，如梧桐子大。每服十丸，饭饮下，温酒下亦得。空心食前服。

Pound the above ingredients into powder, mix with vinegar and make

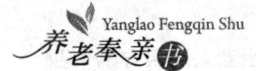

the paste into pills as big as firmiana seeds. Take 10 pills each time with meals or with warm wine. Or take it before meal on an empty stomach.

白香散。治一切恶疮，疼痛不可忍者。

Baixiang San（White Sweetgum Powder）can treat all kinds of malignant ulcers with unbearable pain.

枫香一分，纸衬于地上食顷，令脆，细研　腻粉一分

Prepare one Fen of Fengxiang ［枫香，Chinese Sweetgum, Liquidambar formosana Hance］ and put it on the ground with paper packing, grind finely when it is crispy. Prepare one Fen of calomel.

上二味，同细研令匀。每有患者，先用口内含浆水令暖，吐出洗疮令净后，以药末干傅之，疼痛立止，贴至差为度。

Pound the above ingredients into powder. Warm the mouth and clean the ulcer inside with rice water, apply the powder on the ulcer and the pain can be relieved at once. Apply it like this until the ulcer is healed.

治金疮，水毒，及木签刺，痛疽，热毒等，刻圣散方，金疮此药最妙。

Kesheng San（Powder to Treat Incised Wound）can treat incised wound, damp toxin, hangnail, carbuncles, heat pathogens, etc. It is especially effective to treat incised wound.

糯米三升，拣去粳米，入瓷盆内，于端午日前四十九日，以冷水浸之，以一日两度换水，

轻轻以手淘，转碎去水，勿令搅碎，浸至端午日取出。用干生绢裹，挂于通风处收之

Prepare 3 Sheng of sticky rice, remove the polished round-grained rice, and put it in a porcelain basin. Submerge it in cold water for 49 days before the Dragon Boat Festival and change the water twice a day. Clean it slightly with hands and drain away the water on the Dragon Boat Festival. Wrap it with silk cloth and hang it in a ventilated place.

上旋取少许，炒令焦黑，碾为末，冷水调如膏药大小，裹定疮口外，以绢帛包定，更不要动著，候疮愈。若金疮误犯生水，疮口作脓烘，渐甚者，急以药膏裹定三食久，肿处已消，更不作脓，直至疮合。若痈疽毒疮初发，才觉焮肿赤热，急以膏药贴之，一宿便消。喉闭及咽喉肿痛，吒腮，并用药贴项下及肿处。若竹木签刺入肉者，临卧贴之，明日揭看，其刺出在药内。若贴肿毒，干即换之，常令湿为妙。惟金疮水毒不可换，恐伤疮口发。

Take a little of it and stir-fry until its color becomes dark, crush and mix it with cold water to make it into paste as big as the plaster, apply it on the wound and bandage it with silk cloth, leave it untouched and wait until the wound is healed. If the incised wound accidentally contacts impure water and suppurates with scorching pain, apply the plaster on the wound for the time of taking 3 meals. Then the swelling can be subsided, alongside with the pus removed and the ulcer cured. For the initial onset of ulcer and carbuncle with swelling and heat, apply the plaster on the wound immediately and it will be cured overnight. For pharyngitis, sore throat and mumps, apply the plaster on the neck and the affected area. For piercing wound caused by pegwood, apply the plaster on the wound before sleep and the thorn can be found in the ointment next day. The plaster should be changed to a new one when it is dry for treating swelling, but not changed when treating incised wound to avoid infection.

治手臂疼痛，冷重无力。虎骨散。

Hugu San (Tiger Bone Powder) can treat the pain in the arm, alongside with cold, heaviness, and flaccidity.

虎骨为粗末，炒黄，二钱　羚羊角屑二两　芍药二两

Prepare 2 Qian of Hugu [虎骨, Tiger Bone, Panthera tigris L] pounded into rough powder and stir-fried to brown, 2 Liang of scraps of the Lingyangjiao [羚羊角, Antelope Horn, Cornu Saigae Tataricae], and 2 Liang of Shaoyao [芍药, Paeony, Paeonia lactiflora Pall].

上，一处酒浸一宿，焙，杵为末。每服二钱，食前暖酒调下。

Steep them in wine for one night, bake and pestle into powder. Take 2 Qian each time with warm wine before meals.

治上焦风热毒疮肿。黄芪散。

Huangqi San (Milkvetch Root Powder) can treat wind-heat toxin and swollen sore in the upper energizer.

黄芪二两　防风一两半　甘草一两，炙

Prepare 2 Liang of Huangqi〔黄芪, Astragals, Radix Astragali seu Hedysari〕, one and a half Liang of Fangfeng〔防风, Anisomeles, Radix Ledebouriellae〕, one Liang of Gancao〔甘草, liquorice, Radix Glycyrrhizae〕stir-fried.

上为末，如茶点服一钱。

Pound the above ingredients into powder, take one Qian each time just like tea drinking.

治风气。神白散。

Shenbai San（Effective White Powder）can be used to treat wind pathogen.

白芷二两　甘草一两

Prepare 2 Liang of Baizhi〔白芷, Angelica, Radix Angelicafe Dahuricae〕and one Liang of Gancao〔甘草, Liquorice, Radix Glycyrrhizae〕.

上锉成骰子大，慢火一处炒令深紫色，勿令焦黑。放地上，出火毒，杵为末。每服一钱半，水八分一盏，姜二片，枣二个，同煎至六分，通口服。如伤寒时疾，去枣姜，却入葱白三寸，豉五十粒，依前服。如人行五七里已来，更服，汗出为妙。

Grind the ingredients into paste as big as dice, bake it with slow fire until its color is deep purple and make sure it is not burnt. Put it on the ground to expel its fire toxin and pestle it into powder. Take one and a half

Qian each time, put 2 slices of ginger and 2 Chinese dates in a cup with 8 Fen of water, decoct until three fourths is left and take all the decoction at one time. For cold damage and epidemic diseases, remove the ginger and Chinese dates, add 3 inches of scallion and 50 pills of Douchi［豆豉，Fermented Soybean, Semen Sojae Preparatum］, and take it in the same way as above. Take the decoction again after the time of walking 5 to 7 Li（1 Li equals 0.31 miles）. It would be more effective if sweating is induced after taking the decoction.

治一切心腹刺痛。应痛丸。

Yingtong Wan（Pain Relieving Pill）can treat all kinds of stabbing pain in the heart and abdomen.

乳香一两　五灵脂一两　没药一两　川乌头二两，去皮、脐

Prepare one Liang of Ruxiang［乳香，Olibanum, Resina Olibani］, one Liang of Wulingzhi［五灵脂，Squirrel's Droppings, Faeces Togopteri］, one Liang of Moyao［没药，Myrrha, Commiphora myrrha Engl.］, and 2 Liang of Chuanwutou［川乌头，Aconite Main Root, AconitumcarmichaeliDebx］ with its skin and navel removed.

上为末，面糊为丸如桐子大。每服熟水吞下二十丸。

Pound the above ingredients into powder, mix with flour paste and make them into pills as big as firmiana seeds. Take 20 pills with boiled water each time.

治赤白痢方：

Formula for dealing with red and white dysentery.

黄连半两　汉椒一两

Prepare half a Liang of Huanglian ［黄连，Coptis Root, Rhizoma Coptidis］ and one Liang of Hanjiao ［汉椒，Pepper Fruit, Fructus Piperis Nigri］.

上同炒令黄色，去火毒，为末。以多年水梅肉丸，如绿豆大。每服二十丸，盐汤下。小儿加减用之。

Fry them until they are brown in color to remove the fire toxin, pound them into powder and make them into pills together with the pulp of the aged Wumei ［乌梅，Dark Plum Fruit, Fructus Mume］ as big as mung beans. Take twenty pills each time with salt soup. The dosage for children should be modified accordingly.

养老奉亲书续添

Supplementation

年老丰肥之人，承暑冒热，腹内火烧，遍身汗流，心中焦渴。忽遇冰雪冷浆，尽力而饮，承凉而睡，久而停滞。秋来，不疟则痢。

For the elderly with heavy weight, they are likely to suffer from abdominal fever, heavy sweating, severe thirst due to summer heat in summer days. If they drink cold beverage at will and sleep in cold places, they may suffer from malaria or dysentery due to cold stagnation in the following autumn.

年老丰肥之人，不可骑马，恐有坠堕。宜别置乘座器具，稳当无失。

The elderly with heavy weight shouldn't ride on horses to avoid falling injury. They should take safer vehicles that are stable and reliable.

老人目暗耳聋，肾水衰而心火盛也。若峻补之，则肾水弥涸，心火弥茂。

The elderly are weak in eyesight and hearing due to kidney deficiency and exuberance of heart fire. Drastic tonification will consume kidney water and lead to exuberance of heart fire.

老人肾虚无力，夜多小溲。肾主足，肾水虚而火不下，故足痿；心火上乘肺而不入脬囊，故夜多小溲。若峻补之，则火益上行，脬囊亦寒矣。

The elderly tend to suffer from frequent urination at night due to kidney deficiency and flaccidity. Kidney governs feet and kidney deficiency prevents fire from coordinating with kidney water, resulting in feet flaccidity. The heart fire goes up to subjugate the lung instead of warming the bladder, resulting in frequent urination at night. Drastic tonification will accelerate the fire going upward and worsen the coldness of the bladder.

老人喘嗽，火乘肺也。若温补之则宜，峻补之则危。

The cough of the elderly is caused by fire in the lung, which can be treated and tonified moderately instead of drastically tonification.

老人脏腑结燥，大便秘涩，可频服猪羊血，或葵菜血脏羹，皆能疏利。

The constipation of the elderly due to dryness in the zang-fu organs can be treated by taking pig blood and goat blood, or thick soup made of mallow and animal offal. They are effective to relax the bowel.

老人可常服杏汤，杏仁板儿炒熟，麻子芝麻作汤。服之，亦能通利。

The elderly is suggested to take apricot soup, which is composed of fried almond, flaxseed and sesame, to purge the bowel and move the stool.